HUG ME CLOSE
THE ART OF HUGGING

DIPAN KUMAR DAS

SUDIP KUMAR DAS

To all the hearts that beat with the rhythm of connection, warmth, and understanding,

This book is dedicated to you.

In the spirit of shared embraces and the universal language of hugs, I extend my deepest gratitude to those who have filled the pages of their lives with the art of hugging. To the individuals who have welcomed this exploration into the tender territory of human connection, may the lessons learned within these pages ripple through your own embraces, enriching the tapestry of your relationships.

To the countless souls who have found solace, joy, and healing in the simple yet profound act of hugging, this dedication is a tribute to your resilience, vulnerability, and the enduring capacity of the human heart to connect.

May the warmth of each hug shared within these chapters be reflected in the embraces you extend to others, creating a world where the art of hugging becomes a cherished practice—an art that knows no bounds and serves as a beacon of love and understanding.

With heartfelt appreciation and warm embraces.

Foreword

In the pages that follow, you are about to embark on a journey into the heart of one of the most fundamental aspects of human existence—the art of hugging. As I stand on the precipice of introducing you to this exploration, I am reminded of the profound truth that lies within the simplicity of an embrace.

In a world often marked by the frenetic pace of modern life, the significance of human connection can be easily overlooked. Yet, it is in the warmth of a hug that we find a timeless and universal language—a language that communicates understanding, compassion, and the shared essence of our humanity.

"Hug Me Close: The Art of Hugging" is not just a book; it is an invitation to rediscover the power of touch, to explore the myriad ways in which hugging transcends cultural, generational, and technological boundaries. The artistry of hugging is not bound by words; it is woven into the fabric of our emotions, creating a symphony of connection that resonates with the very essence of who we are.

As you navigate through the chapters that follow, allow yourself to be immersed in the stories, insights, and reflections on the transformative nature of hugs. Whether you are a seasoned hug enthusiast or a newcomer to the world of intentional embraces, I invite you to open your heart to the possibility that lies within each page.

Embrace the art of hugging as not just a physical gesture but as a profound expression of human connection—one that has the power to heal, uplift, and foster a sense of belonging. May this exploration leave you with a renewed appreciation for the warmth that hugs bring to our lives, and may it inspire you to weave the art of hugging into the very fabric of your existence.

With open arms and warm wishes.

Preface

In the dance of life, there exists an unseen thread that binds us all—the thread of connection. This thread weaves through our shared experiences, forming the intricate tapestry of human relationships. As we stand on the threshold of "Hug Me Close: The Art of Hugging," this preface serves as a gentle guide into the heart of our exploration.

In the busyness of our modern world, where screens often mediate our interactions, the significance of physical touch and its emotional resonance can be easily overlooked. This book is an endeavour to unravel the layers of the age-old art of hugging—an art that extends beyond the surface, beyond cultural boundaries, and beyond the constraints of time.

The preface invites you to reflect on the power of touch, the warmth of embraces, and the transformative potential of intentional hugging. Within these pages, you will find stories that resonate with the universal language of hugs, insights into the therapeutic dimensions of embraces, and guidance on navigating the diverse landscapes of hugging culture.

As you turn the pages, allow yourself to be enveloped in the comforting embrace of shared experiences and the exploration of an art form that transcends generations, cultures, and technologies. Consider this book not just as a guide but as a companion on your journey to rediscover the profound beauty that lies within the simple act of hugging.

May the preface serve as an opening chapter to a world where connections are nurtured, where the art of hugging becomes a celebration of our shared humanity, and where the unseen thread of connection is recognized and embraced with open hearts.

With anticipation and warmth.

Prologue

In the quiet spaces between heartbeats, there exists an ancient rhythm—a rhythm that has echoed through the corridors of time. It is the rhythm of the embrace, the silent language of connection that transcends the boundaries of history and culture. As we step into the prologue of "Hug Me Close: The Art of Hugging," we embark on a journey that unravels the timeless tapestry of human connection.

In the prologue, we invite you to imagine the first embrace—the primal gesture that marked the dawn of human existence. Picture the warmth of a comforting hug shared among our ancestors, a gesture born not out of necessity but from an innate understanding of the power held within the touch of another.

As we traverse the epochs, the prologue sets the stage for an exploration into the significance of hugging across civilizations, civilizations that may have crumbled to dust but left behind the indelible imprint of their embrace. Consider this prologue as an invitation to witness the echoes of embraces shared in eras long past, recognizing that the art of hugging is an ancient dance that continues to unfold in the present moment.

Prepare to immerse yourself in the stories of embraces that have shaped history, from the tender gestures exchanged in times of triumph to the solace found in the arms of loved ones during moments of sorrow. The prologue serves as a prelude to the diverse chapters that follow—a reminder that the art of hugging is not just an expression; it is a legacy woven into the very fabric of our shared human experience.

As you embark on this odyssey through time and connection, may the prologue kindle a sense of wonder for the embrace that has endured across millennia, leaving an indomitable mark on the human soul.

7.

Hugging in The Digital Age

8.

Conclusion: The Enduring Warmth of Hugs

Epilogue

CHAPTER ONE

Embracing the Power of Touch

In the quiet corners of our existence, where words often fall short, touch emerges as a profound language, speaking directly to the essence of our humanity. In "Hug Me Close: The Art of Hugging," we embark on a journey that unravels the enchanting world of touch, beginning with the opening chapter – "Embracing the Power of Touch."

The Craving for Connection:

As social beings, the yearning for connection is woven into the fabric of our being. In this chapter, we explore the innate human desire for physical closeness and delve into the roots of why touch holds such sway over our emotions. Drawing from neuroscience and psychology, we unravel the intricate dance between touch and the release of oxytocin, the "love hormone," examining how this biochemical reaction fosters feelings of trust, security, and belonging.

In the intricate tapestry of human existence, the desire for connection is a fundamental thread that binds us together. As social beings, our yearning for interpersonal bonds is deeply ingrained in our nature. This chapter embarks on a journey to unravel the profound significance of physical closeness and explores the roots of why touch has a profound impact on our emotions.

Drawing upon insights from neuroscience and psychology, we aim to decode the complex dance between human touch and the release of oxytocin, often referred to as the "love hormone." Oxytocin, a neuropeptide produced in the brain, plays a pivotal role in shaping our social and emotional experiences.

At its core, the release of oxytocin is intimately tied to our experiences of touch. Whether it be a warm embrace, a gentle hand on the shoulder, or a tender kiss, these physical interactions trigger a cascade of biochemical reactions within our brains. Understanding this intricate interplay sheds light on why touch holds such sway over our emotions.

As we delve into the neurological aspects, we uncover how oxytocin fosters feelings of trust, security, and belonging. This biochemical reaction acts as a powerful bonding agent, creating a sense of connection between individuals. It goes beyond mere physical contact; it is a mechanism that deepens our social bonds and reinforces our sense of community.

Throughout the exploration of the "love hormone," we navigate the profound impact of oxytocin on our mental and emotional well-being. Beyond its role in social bonding, oxytocin has been linked to stress reduction, improved mood, and increased feelings of empathy. This chapter aims to paint a comprehensive picture of how our biological makeup intertwines with our innate desire for connection.

In essence, the intricate dance between touch and the release of oxytocin serves as a testament to the profound interconnectedness of our physical and emotional worlds. As we unravel the mysteries of this biochemical symphony, we gain a deeper understanding of why the yearning for connection is an integral part of what makes us human. Through this exploration, we embark on a journey to recognize, appreciate, and nurture the essential role that touch plays in shaping our relationships and enhancing the tapestry of our shared human experience.

A Symphony of Emotions:

From the tender hug shared between friends to the gentle touch that mends a broken heart, touch serves as a conduit for a myriad of emotions. Through real-life stories and scientific insights, we navigate the emotional landscape that hugs traverse, understanding how they can communicate joy, empathy, and solace without the need for words. This chapter aims to illuminate the transformative power of touch in cultivating emotional well-being.

The power of touch in human interactions is a profound and multifaceted aspect of our lives. From the simplest gestures like a handshake to more intimate expressions such as a hug, touch plays a crucial role in conveying emotions and fostering connections. This chapter delves into the emotional landscape that hugs, in particular, traverse, shedding light on their ability to communicate joy, empathy, and solace in ways that words often fall short.

Real-life stories serve as poignant examples of how touch can be a powerful means of communication. The tender hug shared between friends illustrates the warmth and support that can be conveyed without the need for verbal expressions. In times of joy, a hug can amplify the shared happiness, creating a tangible and visceral connection that goes beyond spoken language.

Conversely, the gentle touch that mends a broken heart speaks to the soothing and healing properties of physical contact. Scientific insights into the neurobiology of touch reveal that physical interactions, such as hugs, release oxytocin, often referred to as the "love hormone" or "bonding hormone." This hormone is associated with social bonding, trust, and emotional well-being, providing a biological basis for the emotional impact of touch.

Understanding the transformative power of touch is essential in recognizing its role in cultivating emotional well-being. The tactile experiences we share with others contribute to a sense of belonging and emotional connection. In times of distress, a comforting touch can convey empathy and offer solace, providing a profound form of emotional support.

As we navigate the intricate tapestry of human emotions, it becomes evident that touch serves as a conduit for a myriad of feelings. Whether it's a celebratory embrace or a consoling touch, these physical interactions contribute significantly to our overall emotional health. By acknowledging and appreciating the transformative power of touch, we gain a deeper understanding of its role in fostering meaningful connections and promoting emotional well-being.

The Science Behind the Hug:

At its core, the art of hugging is deeply rooted in science. This section of the chapter takes readers on a captivating exploration of the physiological effects of touch on the human body. From the regulation of stress hormones to the enhancement of immune function, we uncover the myriad ways in which hugging contributes to our overall health. The reader will gain a newfound appreciation for the intricate dance between touch and well-being.

In the realm of human connection, the seemingly simple act of a hug emerges as a powerful force, with its roots intricately woven into the fabric of science. This section of the chapter endeavors to unravel the physiological effects of touch, specifically focusing on the profound impact that hugging has on the human body.

At the forefront of this exploration is the regulation of stress hormones. Hugging, it turns out, is not merely a comforting gesture; it is a potent stress-reliever. When we engage in a warm embrace, our bodies respond by reducing the production of stress hormones, such as cortisol. This physiological response is a crucial component of the intricate dance between touch and our overall well-being. Understanding how a hug can act as a natural stress-reduction mechanism underscores the significance of this simple yet profound gesture.

Beyond stress regulation, the act of hugging has been linked to the enhancement of immune function. Research suggests that regular physical touch, including hugging, can contribute to a strengthened immune system. The mechanisms behind this phenomenon are multifaceted, involving the intricate interplay of neurotransmitters, hormones, and the overall balance of the body's physiological processes. As we delve into the science behind the hug, we gain insights into how these physical interactions can positively impact our health on a systemic level.

Furthermore, the release of oxytocin, often referred to as the "love hormone," is a key player in the science behind the hug. As explored in the previous section, oxytocin fosters feelings of trust, security, and belonging. In the context of hugging, the release of oxytocin contributes not only to emotional bonding but also to the regulation of various physiological processes. This hormonal cascade, triggered by the simple act of a hug, exemplifies the intricate connection between touch and overall well-being.

As readers embark on this captivating exploration, they will gain a newfound appreciation for the profound ways in which hugging contributes to our health. The science behind the hug unveils a holistic perspective on the interconnectedness of our physical and emotional experiences. It reinforces the notion that the desire for connection goes beyond a mere social construct; it is deeply ingrained in our biology, shaping our health and enriching the tapestry of our human experience.

Beyond Words: The Silent Language of Touch:

In a world saturated with communication, touch remains a silent language that often speaks louder than words. This section delves into the nuances of non-verbal communication through touch, exploring how a simple embrace can convey understanding, compassion, and support. Readers will learn to decipher the silent language of touch, recognizing its ability to bridge gaps and create profound connections.

In the cacophony of verbal communication that defines our world, touch emerges as a profound and silent language that often communicates more eloquently than words ever could. This section of the chapter delves into the intricate nuances of non-verbal communication through touch, unraveling the ways in which a simple embrace can convey understanding, compassion, and unwavering support.

In the realm of human interaction, touch has the power to transcend linguistic barriers, cultural differences, and even emotional complexities. It is a universal language that speaks directly to our shared human experience. Through a gentle touch, we can express empathy, convey solace, and forge connections that go beyond the limitations of spoken language.

The silent language of touch becomes particularly poignant when words fail to capture the depth of our emotions or when we find ourselves in situations where verbal communication is challenging. A comforting touch during times of grief, a reassuring hand on the shoulder in moments of uncertainty, or a warm embrace that conveys unspoken solidarity - these gestures communicate a myriad of emotions that often elude verbal expression.

Readers will embark on a journey to decipher the silent language of touch, recognizing its capacity to bridge gaps and create profound connections. It is a form of communication that taps into the primal, instinctual aspects of our humanity, fostering understanding and empathy on a visceral level.

As we explore the silent language of touch, we uncover its ability to convey complex emotions, build trust, and strengthen relationships. This section invites readers to reflect on their own experiences with touch, encouraging an appreciation for the subtle yet potent ways in which physical connection enhances the richness of our interactions.

In a world where words can be misinterpreted or fall short, the silent language of touch stands as a testament to the profound communicative power inherent in our tactile experiences. Through this exploration, readers will gain a deeper understanding of the unspoken connections forged through touch and the transformative impact of this silent language on the human experience.

The Fundamental Role of Hugging in Human Connection:

As we progress through this chapter, the reader is invited to perceive the art of hugging not merely as a casual physical interaction but as a fundamental aspect of human connection. We dissect the layers of significance that hugs add to our relationships, friendships, and familial bonds. Through this exploration, readers will start to appreciate the deep-rooted role that hugging plays in fostering meaningful connections.

Hugging, often seen as a simple and commonplace gesture, holds a profound significance in human connection. This chapter invites the reader to transcend the notion of hugging as a casual physical interaction and instead view it as a fundamental aspect of our relationships, friendships, and familial bonds. By dissecting the layers of significance that hugs contribute to these connections, we aim to shed light on the deep-rooted role that hugging plays in fostering meaningful and authentic human connections.

Hugs go beyond the physical act; they are a language of their own, capable of expressing a range of emotions and sentiments without uttering a single word. In the exploration of the art of hugging, we unravel the layers of meaning that accompany different types of embraces. Whether it's a tight squeeze between loved ones, a comforting pat on the back, or a gentle embrace during a vulnerable moment, each form of hug communicates a unique message that resonates on an emotional level.

Through this journey, readers will gain a heightened awareness of how hugging contributes to the fabric of our relationships. We delve into the physiological and psychological aspects of hugging, exploring the release of oxytocin, the bonding hormone, and its impact on our emotional well-being. This understanding adds depth to the appreciation of hugging as more than just a physical act but as a mechanism that strengthens the bonds between individuals.

Moreover, we examine cultural and societal perspectives on hugging, recognizing its universal appeal while respecting individual preferences and boundaries. As readers navigate through the exploration of hugging, they will start to recognize its role in building trust, creating a sense of security, and fostering intimacy in various relationships.

By the end of this chapter, the reader is encouraged to appreciate the nuanced and fundamental role that hugging plays in the intricate tapestry of human connection. Hugging becomes more than a reflexive response; it becomes a deliberate and meaningful act that enhances the quality of our relationships, ultimately contributing to a deeper sense of belonging, understanding, and emotional fulfillment.

In "Hug Me Close: The Art of Hugging," this opening chapter serves as a gateway into the exploration of touch – a journey that promises to unveil the intricate tapestry of human connection woven through the simple, yet powerful, act of embracing one another.

CHAPTER TWO

The Language of Hugs

In the intricate dance of human connection, hugs emerge as a silent language, a form of communication that transcends the barriers of words. As we continue our exploration in "Hug Me Close: The Art of Hugging," we enter Chapter 2, where the subtle nuances of this language unfold in a myriad of embraces.

The Comforting Bear Hug:

Our journey begins with the iconic bear hug – a warm, enveloping embrace that speaks volumes in its intensity. This section delves into the comforting power of the bear hug, dissecting its ability to convey solace, empathy, and unwavering support. Through anecdotes and insights, readers will grasp the significance of this hug style in fostering a sense of security and reassurance.

In the quiet haven of a moonlit night, beneath a sky adorned with a tapestry of twinkling stars, there existed a realm of solace known to those who sought respite from the chaos of the world. In this tranquil sanctuary, a phenomenon unfolded, a phenomenon known as "The Comforting Bear Hug."

Nestled within the heart of a mystical forest, where ancient trees whispered tales of time, a gentle bear, wise beyond measure, stood sentinel. This bear, adorned in a coat of the softest fur imaginable, emanated an aura of warmth and understanding. Its eyes sparkled with kindness, reflecting the compassion that dwelled within.

Word had spread among the woodland creatures about the magical embrace this bear offered to any weary soul seeking solace. Those who sought comfort would make their way through the rustling leaves and dappled moonlight until they arrived at the clearing where the bear patiently awaited.

As one approached, the bear would raise its massive yet tender arms, inviting the weary traveler into an embrace that transcended the physical realm. The comforting bear hug was no ordinary hug; it was a fusion of empathy, understanding, and a silent promise that, within this moment, all troubles would dissipate.

With a gentle squeeze, the bear's embrace radiated a soothing energy that enveloped the troubled heart and calmed the restless mind. The worries of the world melted away, leaving only the serenity of the present moment. In the comforting bear hug, time seemed to stand still, allowing the recipient to find solace in the simple act of being held.

The mystical forest echoed with the whispers of gratitude as each visitor departed, carrying with them a renewed spirit and a heart lightened by the weight of the world. The comforting bear hug became a symbol of sanctuary, a refuge for those in need of reassurance, and a reminder that, even in the vastness of the universe, there exists a haven where warmth and understanding embrace all who seek it.

Embarking on our exploration of the profound world of human connection, we find ourselves enveloped in the timeless embrace of the bear hug – a gesture that transcends words, reaching deep into the realm of emotions. Picture a moment when you, perhaps weary or distressed, were met with the open arms of a friend or loved one. The bear hug, with its warm, all-encompassing grip, has a unique ability to convey solace and understanding.

This section aims to unravel the layers of comfort woven into the fabric of a bear hug, examining how this simple yet powerful gesture speaks volumes in its intensity.

Through anecdotes and insights, we will uncover the subtle nuances that make the bear hug a universally recognized symbol of empathy and unwavering support.

At its core, the bear hug is a physical manifestation of emotional connection. It goes beyond the surface, allowing individuals to share a moment of vulnerability without uttering a single word. In the warmth of the embrace, there lies a language of reassurance that transcends cultural and linguistic boundaries. It is a universal dialect of compassion, where the arms become conduits of understanding and empathy.

Consider the times when life's challenges seemed insurmountable – a loss, a setback, or even a day that left you emotionally drained. In those moments, a bear hug acts as a silent declaration that you are not alone. The comforting pressure of the arms around you serves as a shield against the storms of life, offering a sanctuary where troubles momentarily fade away.

The bear hug is a testament to the power of touch in fostering a sense of security. Psychologically, it releases oxytocin – the "love hormone" – promoting feelings of trust and bonding. As we delve into personal stories and shared experiences, readers will come to appreciate how this embrace, with its genuine warmth, acts as a bridge connecting hearts and alleviating the burdens of the soul.

Whether between friends, family members, or romantic partners, the bear hug is a versatile expression of love and support. Its impact extends far beyond the physical realm, influencing emotional well-being and creating lasting memories. In the comforting embrace of the bear hug, we find a timeless reminder that, in the ebb and flow of life, there exists a refuge in the arms of those who care.

The Gentle Squeeze of Reassurance:

Moving from the grandeur of the bear hug, we transition to the gentle squeeze – a subtle yet powerful gesture of reassurance. This part of the chapter explores how a delicate, supportive squeeze communicates understanding and encouragement. Readers will discover the art of providing solace through a touch that whispers, "I'm here for you," without uttering a single word.

Transitioning from the grandeur of the bear hug, we now enter the realm of the gentle squeeze – a nuanced yet potent gesture that speaks volumes in its subtlety. In this part of the chapter, we embark on an exploration of how a delicate, supportive squeeze conveys profound reassurance, unveiling the art of providing solace through a touch that whispers, "I'm here for you," without the need for words.

Unlike the all-encompassing nature of the bear hug, the gentle squeeze is characterized by its finesse. It is a touch that transcends the physical, reaching into the emotional landscape with a gentle yet unmistakable presence. As we delve into this section, readers will unravel the intricacies of this understated gesture and understand how it forms a unique language of understanding and encouragement.

Imagine a moment of vulnerability, where words falter in capturing the depth of emotion. It is in these instances that the gentle squeeze finds its place – a quiet reassurance that transcends verbal communication. It is a touch that says, "I acknowledge your struggle, and I am here to support you." In its subtlety, the gentle squeeze becomes an unspoken promise of solidarity.

This part of the chapter delves into personal anecdotes and shared experiences, illustrating how the gentle squeeze serves as a lifeline during challenging times. Whether it's a friend facing uncertainty, a family member navigating a difficult decision, or a partner grappling with insecurities, the gentle squeeze becomes a silent pact that communicates empathy and unwavering support.

The power of the gentle squeeze lies not only in its simplicity but in its ability to create a bridge of connection between individuals. It is a touch that fosters a sense of trust and understanding, allowing for a shared emotional experience. Readers will come to appreciate the elegance of this gesture and its capacity to offer solace in moments where words fall short.

As we navigate through stories that unfold the impact of the gentle squeeze, a deeper understanding will emerge of how this subtle yet powerful gesture contributes to the tapestry of human connection. It is a reminder that in the symphony of relationships, sometimes the most comforting notes are the ones played with a gentle touch – a squeeze that echoes, "I am here, and you are not alone."

Cultural Expressions of Affection:

Hugs are a universal language, but they come adorned with cultural nuances that add a unique flavor to their expression. In this section, we traverse the globe, exploring how different cultures communicate affection through their distinct styles of hugging. From the warm embrace of the Mediterranean to the polite cheek-to-cheek hug in many European countries, readers gain insight into the rich tapestry of hugging traditions worldwide.

Hugs, as a universal language of human connection, take on diverse and culturally enriched forms that weave a colorful tapestry across the globe. This section invites readers on a journey around the world, exploring the myriad ways in which different cultures express affection through their unique styles of hugging. From the warm embrace of the Mediterranean to the polite cheek-to-cheek hug in many European countries, we delve into the rich variety of hugging traditions that reflect the cultural diversity of human relationships.

The Mediterranean region, known for its vibrant and expressive culture, boasts a style of hugging that is as warm as its climate. Here, hugs are not just gestures but heartfelt expressions, often accompanied by a series of kisses on both cheeks. This tactile embrace transcends mere greeting; it is a celebration of connection, a testament to the importance of personal bonds in Mediterranean societies.

In many European countries, the cheek-to-cheek hug is a common practice, showcasing a blend of politeness and intimacy. This form of hugging involves a gentle touch of cheeks while maintaining a certain level of personal space, creating a harmonious balance between warmth and decorum. Each embrace becomes a choreography of cultural etiquette, expressing affection without crossing cultural boundaries.

Across Asia, hugging traditions vary significantly. In some Eastern cultures, such as Japan, hugs may be perceived as more reserved, with a preference for bows or other non-contact forms of greeting. However, in other parts of Asia, like India, warm and familial hugs are integral to expressing love and camaraderie.

African cultures often embrace hugging as a deeply symbolic act. Hugs can signify unity, community, and shared experiences. In many African societies, the warmth of a hug is not limited to individuals but extends to the community at large, fostering a sense of togetherness and belonging.

Exploring the Americas unveils a spectrum of hugging customs. In Latin American countries, passionate and affectionate embraces are common, reflecting the region's vibrant and emotionally expressive culture. In North America, the one-armed hug or "bro hug" is a popular style among friends, combining a handshake with a casual side hug.

As we traverse the continents, readers will gain a richer understanding of how cultural nuances shape the way affection is communicated through hugs. Each cultural expression adds a unique flavor to the universal language of hugs, creating a beautiful mosaic that reflects the intricate dance of human connection across the world.

The Nuanced Meanings Behind Hug Styles:

Beyond cultural differences, the art of hugging reveals a nuanced language where each style carries its own set of meanings. This part of the chapter decodes the unspoken messages behind various hug styles, from the quick pat on the back to the lingering embrace. Readers will learn to navigate the intricacies of this non-verbal language, understanding how subtle variations in hugs can convey friendship, love, or support.

Diving deeper into the art of hugging, we uncover a nuanced language where each style carries its own set of meanings, transcending cultural differences. In this section of the chapter, we embark on a journey to decode the unspoken messages behind various hug styles. From the quick pat on the back to the lingering embrace, readers will gain insight into the subtle variations of this non-verbal language, learning how hugs communicate friendship, love, or support.

The Quick Pat: A seemingly simple gesture, the quick pat on the back is often associated with casual or friendly encounters. It's the type of hug you might share with a colleague or an acquaintance, conveying warmth without delving too deeply into emotional intimacy. The rhythmic pat serves as a friendly punctuation mark, keeping the interaction light and easy-going.

The Side Hug: A familiar sight among friends or acquaintances, the side hug is characterized by its partial embrace, with one arm around the other person. It strikes a balance between warmth and informality, expressing a connection without fully entering the realm of personal space. Common among friends, this hug style signals camaraderie and shared experiences.

The Bear Hug: As explored earlier, the bear hug is a grand, all-encompassing embrace that conveys deep affection and unwavering support. Often shared among close friends or family members, this hug style symbolizes a profound connection, offering solace and reassurance in times of need.

The Linger: A hug that extends beyond the typical duration may carry additional layers of meaning. The lingering embrace often signifies a desire for closeness and emotional connection. Whether between romantic partners or close friends, this style suggests a reluctance to let go, emphasizing the importance of the bond shared.

The Cheek-to-Cheek Hug: This style, common in many European countries, involves a gentle touch of cheeks and expresses a blend of politeness and intimacy. It suggests a level of familiarity and connection, but with a cultural emphasis on maintaining personal space. It conveys warmth while adhering to social norms of decorum.

The One-Armed Hug or "Bro Hug": Frequently seen among friends, particularly in North America, the one-armed hug combines a handshake with a casual side hug. This style suggests a comfortable camaraderie, blending the formality of a handshake with the informality of a hug, making it suitable for both social and professional settings.

Understanding the nuanced meanings behind hug styles empowers readers to navigate the intricate landscape of non-verbal communication. Each hug, whether brief or lingering, conveys a unique message, allowing individuals to express emotions and connections in a language that surpasses the need for words. As we unravel the intricacies of these embraces, we gain a deeper appreciation for the multifaceted art of hugging.

Expressing Emotions through Hug Styles:

As we progress, the chapter delves into the emotional spectrum of hug styles. From the exuberant greeting hug to the tender farewell embrace, readers will explore how different emotions find expression through hugging. This section serves as a guide for readers to recognize and reciprocate the emotions conveyed in various hug styles, fostering deeper connections through shared experiences.

Continuing our exploration, this chapter delves into the emotional spectrum of hug styles, unraveling the various ways in which different emotions find expression through physical embrace. From the exuberant greeting hug to the tender farewell embrace, readers will embark on a journey to understand how the language of hugs becomes a powerful tool for conveying and reciprocating emotions. This section serves as a guide, enabling readers to recognize and respond to the emotions conveyed in diverse hug styles, ultimately fostering deeper connections through shared experiences.

The Exuberant Greeting Hug: Picture the joyous reunion of old friends or loved ones separated by time and distance. The exuberant greeting hug is characterized by its enthusiasm, often involving laughter, spinning, or even a lifting off the ground. This hug style is a celebration of happiness and shared moments, expressing an overwhelming sense of joy and connection.

The Comforting Sympathy Hug: In times of sorrow or distress, the comforting sympathy hug serves as a lifeline of support. This embrace is characterized by its tenderness, offering solace and reassurance to those experiencing hardship. The slow, soothing movements convey empathy and an unwavering commitment to being there for someone in need.

The Electric Romantic Hug: Shared between romantic partners, the electric romantic hug is charged with passion and desire. It goes beyond the conventional embrace, often involving a lingering touch, a gentle caress, or an intimate closeness. This style speaks the language of love, expressing desire, and building an emotional connection between partners.

The Heartfelt Gratitude Hug: When words fall short in expressing gratitude, the heartfelt gratitude hug steps in. This embrace is sincere and earnest, conveying appreciation and thankfulness. Whether it's acknowledging a supportive friend, a mentor, or someone who made a difference, this hug style communicates a depth of gratitude that goes beyond verbal expression.

The Nostalgic Reunion Hug: Reconnecting with someone from the past often evokes a mix of emotions. The nostalgic reunion hug encapsulates a sense of familiarity, nostalgia, and perhaps a touch of sentimentality. It's a hug that bridges the gap between past and present, expressing the joy of rediscovery.

The Tender Farewell Hug: Parting ways, whether temporarily or permanently, is an emotional moment that the tender farewell hug encapsulates. This hug style is marked by its gentleness, conveying love, and a sense of longing. It serves as a poignant farewell, expressing emotions that words alone cannot capture.

Recognizing and reciprocating the emotions embedded in each hug style allows individuals to navigate the intricate landscape of human connections more effectively. This section of the chapter encourages readers to not only understand the emotional undertones of hugs but also to embrace the opportunity to share these emotions with others, fostering deeper and more meaningful relationships through the universal language of touch.

Creating Personalized Hug Traditions:

The chapter concludes by encouraging readers to embrace the art of creating personalized hug traditions. By understanding the language of hugs, individuals can cultivate their own unique styles of embracing, fostering a more intimate and authentic form of communication in their relationships. Through this exploration, readers will gain a deeper understanding of how to express themselves and connect with others through the language of hugs.

As we draw the chapter to a close, readers are invited to embark on the art of creating personalized hug traditions. By delving into the nuanced language of hugs explored throughout this journey, individuals can cultivate their own unique styles of embracing, fostering a more intimate and authentic form of communication in their relationships. This exploration aims to empower readers with a deeper understanding of how to express themselves and connect with others through the personalized and universal language of hugs.

The beauty of personalized hug traditions lies in their authenticity and ability to reflect the unique dynamics of each relationship. Whether among friends, family, or romantic partners, individuals can infuse their hugs with personal meaning, creating rituals that go beyond the conventional. This could involve the development of specific gestures, like a secret handshake combined with a hug, or even the establishment of certain phrases that accompany the embrace.

Consider incorporating elements that resonate with shared experiences or inside jokes, turning each hug into a testament of the journey shared. Personalized hug traditions become a mirror of the connection between individuals, encapsulating the essence of their relationship in a physical gesture. This not only deepens the bond but also allows for the expression of emotions in a way that is uniquely theirs.

Experimentation is key in crafting these personalized hug traditions. Trying different styles, exploring variations in duration, and paying attention to the emotional context of each embrace can contribute to the evolution of a meaningful and personalized hugging ritual. The process of co-creating these traditions can itself become a bonding experience, fostering a sense of collaboration and understanding.

In this concluding section, readers are encouraged to reflect on their own relationships and consider how the language of hugs can be uniquely tailored to express their emotions and strengthen their connections. By embracing the art of personalized hug traditions, individuals not only communicate more authentically but also contribute to the enrichment of their relationships through a shared and cherished form of expression.

In essence, the journey through the diverse hug styles, cultural expressions, and emotional nuances explored in this chapter serves as an inspiration for readers to go beyond the conventional and create their own tapestry of hug traditions. In doing so, they contribute to the ever-evolving language of human connection, where each embrace becomes a chapter in the story of shared experiences, emotions, and the enduring power of touch.

In "Hug Me Close: The Art of Hugging," Chapter 2 opens the door to a world where every embrace is a conversation, and the language of hugs becomes a guide to more meaningful connections.

CHAPTER THREE

The Therapeutic Hug

As we venture deeper into the heart of "Hug Me Close: The Art of Hugging," Chapter 3 beckons us into the transformative realm of therapeutic hugs. In this chapter, we unravel the profound impact that embraces can have on our mental and emotional well-being, transcending their role as mere gestures of affection.

The Healing Power of Touch:

At the core of therapeutic hugging lies the recognition that touch possesses an extraordinary ability to heal. Drawing from scientific research, we explore the neurobiological mechanisms that underlie the therapeutic effects of hugs. From the release of endorphins to the reduction of cortisol levels, readers will gain insights into how the simple act of embracing can be a potent antidote to stress and anxiety.

In the intricate dance of human connection, therapeutic hugging emerges as a profound testament to the healing power of touch. Beyond its surface-level expressions, touch carries an innate ability to weave threads of comfort, empathy, and understanding into the fabric of our well-being. Delving into the realms of science, we uncover the intricate neurobiological mechanisms that illuminate the therapeutic effects of hugs, casting light on the profound impact that this simple act can have on our mental and emotional states.

At the heart of the matter lies the release of endorphins, often referred to as the body's natural feel-good chemicals. Scientific studies have shown that the gentle pressure and warmth experienced during a hug stimulate the production of these neurotransmitters, creating a cascade of positive effects. Endorphins not only act as natural painkillers but also play a crucial role in alleviating stress and promoting an overall sense of well-being.

Furthermore, the act of hugging has been linked to the reduction of cortisol levels, the hormone associated with stress. Cortisol, when released in excess, can contribute to a range of health issues, from anxiety to sleep disturbances. Through the comforting embrace of a hug, the body's stress response is tempered, leading to a decrease in cortisol production and fostering a state of relaxation.

The therapeutic benefits of touch extend beyond the biochemical realm, reaching into the intricacies of human connection and emotional support. Hugging has been found to enhance the release of oxytocin, often referred to as the "love hormone" or "bonding hormone." Oxytocin plays a pivotal role in building and strengthening social bonds, fostering trust, and promoting a sense of security. As we engage in the act of hugging, we not only experience a surge of warmth and connection but also nourish the foundation of our emotional well-being.

In a world where stress and anxiety can often seem inescapable, the simplicity of a hug emerges as a potent antidote. By understanding the neurobiological tapestry woven through the act of embracing, we unravel the profound healing potential embedded within our capacity for touch. Therapeutic hugging becomes a reminder that, amidst the complexities of life, a moment of shared warmth and connection can serve as a powerful balm for the soul, promoting resilience and fortifying the bonds that make us fundamentally human.

Hugging Away Stress:

In this section, we delve into the role of hugs as a natural stress-reliever. Through real-life anecdotes and expert opinions, readers will understand how the physical closeness of a hug triggers a cascade of physiological responses that counteract the effects of stress. From workplace tension to personal challenges, therapeutic hugging emerges as a readily available remedy to navigate the complexities of daily life.

In the hustle and bustle of our modern lives, stress can often become an unwelcome companion, manifesting in various forms and affecting our overall well-being. As we navigate the challenges of work, relationships, and personal growth, the simple yet profound act of hugging emerges as a natural stress-reliever, offering solace and respite from the demands of daily life.

Real-life anecdotes serve as poignant testaments to the transformative power of hugs in alleviating stress. Individuals from diverse backgrounds and walks of life share their experiences of seeking comfort in the embrace of a loved one during moments of tension and pressure. Whether facing workplace challenges or personal hardships, the physical closeness of a hug becomes a source of strength, providing a tangible and immediate response to the stressors that life throws our way.

Experts weigh in on the science behind this phenomenon, shedding light on how the act of hugging triggers a cascade of physiological responses that counteract the effects of stress. As we embrace someone, the sensory receptors in our skin send signals to the brain, activating the release of endorphins - the body's natural stress-busters. Simultaneously, the gentle pressure and warmth of a hug prompt a reduction in cortisol levels, easing the grip of stress on our minds and bodies.

Workplace tension, in particular, is a common battleground for stress, with deadlines, meetings, and interpersonal dynamics contributing to a high-stakes environment. Yet, the power of therapeutic hugging offers a simple and accessible remedy to navigate these complexities. Through anecdotes shared by individuals in professional settings, we explore how the exchange of hugs among colleagues or the supportive embrace of a friend can create a more harmonious and resilient workplace, fostering a sense of camaraderie that transcends professional challenges.

In the realm of personal challenges, whether it be navigating relationship issues or coping with life's uncertainties, hugs emerge as a universal language of comfort and understanding. Realizing the profound impact that physical closeness can have on our mental and emotional states, individuals find solace in the arms of loved ones, creating a haven of support amid life's storms.

As we journey through the complexities of daily life, therapeutic hugging stands as a readily available remedy, a tangible and immediate response to the stresses that threaten to overwhelm us. Through the lens of real-life stories and expert insights, we come to appreciate the extraordinary power of hugs to soothe, heal, and navigate the intricate tapestry of stress that we all weave in our lives.

Embracing Emotional Resilience:

The therapeutic hug extends its reach beyond stress relief to foster emotional resilience. This part of the chapter explores how regular, meaningful embraces contribute to emotional well-being by creating a sense of security and connection. Readers will discover the art of building emotional resilience through the consistent practice of embracing, allowing them to face life's challenges with a strengthened spirit.

As we unravel the multifaceted layers of therapeutic hugging, it becomes evident that its impact transcends the immediate relief of stress. This section delves into the transformative realm of emotional resilience, illuminating how regular and meaningful embraces contribute to a profound sense of well-being, fostering a spirit that can withstand the challenges life presents.

At its core, the therapeutic hug becomes a cornerstone in the construction of emotional resilience by creating a cocoon of security and connection. Through the warmth and comfort of an embrace, individuals experience a profound sense of safety and belonging, reinforcing their emotional fortitude. Real-life stories underscore the enduring power of hugs as individuals navigate the ebbs and flows of life, finding solace in the arms of loved ones during moments of vulnerability.

Experts in psychology and neuroscience provide insights into the intricate dance between touch and emotional resilience. The release of oxytocin, often referred to as the "love hormone," takes center stage, fostering a deep sense of connection and trust. Regular, meaningful embraces contribute to the maintenance of elevated oxytocin levels, nurturing a resilient emotional foundation that allows individuals to confront life's challenges with a strengthened spirit.

The art of building emotional resilience through the consistent practice of embracing becomes apparent, as readers are guided through the journey of integrating therapeutic hugging into their daily lives. Whether facing personal setbacks, relationship challenges, or the inevitable twists and turns of life, the embrace serves as a grounding force, reminding individuals of their capacity to weather storms and emerge stronger on the other side.

In exploring the connection between hugs and emotional resilience, we find that the act of embracing becomes more than a momentary reprieve; it evolves into a proactive strategy for building a resilient mindset. Through the exchange of hugs, individuals not only find comfort in times of need but also cultivate a reservoir of inner strength that becomes a wellspring of resilience when faced with adversity.

As we navigate the labyrinth of emotions and trials, the therapeutic hug emerges as a steadfast ally, offering a sanctuary where emotional resilience is nurtured and fortified. This chapter invites readers to embrace the art of building emotional resilience through the simple yet profound act of hugging, empowering them to face life's challenges with a spirit that is not only unyielding but also capable of finding beauty and growth amidst the complexities of the human experience.

The Comforting Hug as Emotional Medicine:

Beyond the science, we delve into the emotional narratives of individuals who have found solace in the therapeutic embrace. Through poignant stories of healing and renewal, readers will witness how hugs serve as emotional medicine, offering comfort in times of grief, loneliness, or despair. This section highlights the capacity of hugs to provide a safe space for emotional expression and recovery.

In the realm of therapeutic hugging, the profound impact goes beyond the realms of scientific explanations, reaching into the emotional narratives of individuals who have found solace in the comforting embrace. Beyond the clinical analyses, this section unfolds through poignant stories of healing and renewal, illustrating how hugs function as a form of emotional medicine – a source of comfort in times of grief, loneliness, or despair.

Real-life stories become the canvas on which the therapeutic hug paints its most powerful strokes. Readers are invited to witness the transformative journeys of individuals who, in the midst of emotional turmoil, discovered the unparalleled healing potential encapsulated in a simple yet profound hug. These narratives speak to the universal language of human emotions, transcending cultural and societal boundaries, as individuals find refuge in the warm embrace of loved ones during times of distress.

The embrace emerges as a poignant symbol of emotional medicine, offering a balm for wounds that are often invisible to the naked eye. From grief-stricken hearts to those grappling with the isolating tendrils of loneliness, the therapeutic hug becomes a safe harbor for emotional expression and recovery. Through the unspoken language of touch, individuals navigate the complex landscapes of their emotions, finding solace in the understanding and comfort offered by a loved one's arms.

These emotional narratives underscore the capacity of hugs to serve as a sanctuary for vulnerability, a space where individuals can shed the weight of their burdens and allow themselves to be seen and supported. The act of hugging becomes a powerful form of emotional medicine, transcending verbal communication to provide a tangible and immediate response to the deepest recesses of human suffering.

In exploring these stories, readers are invited to reflect on the profound impact of the therapeutic hug on emotional well-being. It becomes evident that, in the face of life's adversities, the embrace serves as a timeless remedy – an emotional medicine that transcends the limitations of language and offers a bridge to healing, renewal, and the restoration of hope. Through the lens of these heartfelt narratives, the comforting hug emerges not just as a physical act but as a beacon of emotional support, reminding us of the extraordinary capacity of human touch to heal and mend the wounds of the soul.

Reconnecting Generations: Sarah, a busy professional, finds herself overwhelmed by the demands of her career and disconnected from her family. A simple family gathering turns into a transformative experience when her grandmother, sensing her distress, offers a warm and lingering hug. In that embrace, Sarah rediscovers a sense of belonging and emotional connection, realizing that the therapeutic hug has the power to bridge generational gaps and provide a timeless source of comfort.

Healing Hearts: Mark, grieving the loss of a loved one, struggles to navigate the waves of sorrow. Amidst the condolences, a friend offers a silent yet profound hug. In that shared moment, Mark feels the weight of his grief lifted ever so slightly. The therapeutic hug becomes a gentle but potent medicine, offering a sanctuary for Mark to express his emotions without words, fostering a path towards healing.

Friendship's Embrace: Emily, facing the challenges of a tumultuous friendship, experiences the emotional rollercoaster of betrayal and confusion. In a pivotal moment, her closest friend reaches out with a comforting hug, transcending the need for words. The therapeutic embrace becomes a bridge of understanding and forgiveness, reminding Emily that the bonds of friendship are resilient and can weather even the stormiest of conflicts.

Parental Comfort: Jake, a teenager navigating the complexities of adolescence, grapples with self-doubt and identity. During a particularly challenging day, his parent offers an understanding and supportive hug. In that moment, Jake discovers that the therapeutic hug serves as a lifeline for adolescents, providing a secure space for them to navigate the turbulent seas of self-discovery and emotional turbulence.

The Healing Circle: In a support group for survivors of trauma, individuals share stories of resilience and recovery. As they recount their experiences, the group discovers the unspoken power of forming a healing circle, where therapeutic hugs become a communal language of empathy and understanding. In this shared embrace, the members find strength, realizing that the therapeutic hug has the capacity to knit together the fragmented pieces of their lives into a tapestry of collective healing.

Incorporating Therapeutic Hugs into Daily Life:

This chapter is not just an exploration but a practical guide. Here, readers will find actionable insights on how to incorporate therapeutic hugs into their daily routines. From mindful hugging exercises to creating a culture of embracing in relationships, this section equips readers with the tools to harness the therapeutic potential of hugs in their own lives.

As we embark on the journey of integrating therapeutic hugs into the fabric of our daily existence, this chapter transcends mere exploration, evolving into a practical guide designed to empower readers with actionable insights. Beyond the theoretical understanding, readers will discover tangible tools and exercises to seamlessly weave the profound therapeutic potential of hugs into the tapestry of their daily lives.

1. Mindful Hugging Exercises: Begin your day with a mindful hugging exercise, setting the tone for emotional well-being. Whether it's a partner, family member, or even a pet, engage in a conscious embrace. Focus on the sensations of touch, the rise and fall of breath, and the warmth exchanged. This intentional practice not only nurtures a sense of connection but also lays the groundwork for a resilient mindset throughout the day.

2. Creating a Culture of Embracing in Relationships: Foster a culture of embracing within your relationships, both romantic and platonic. Communicate openly with your loved ones about the significance of hugs in promoting emotional well-being. Establish a mutual understanding that embraces are not just reserved for moments of distress but are integral to the everyday expression of care and support. Encourage each other to initiate hugs as a spontaneous gesture of connection.

3. The Power of Ritualized Hugging: Integrate ritualized hugging into specific

moments of your routine. Whether it's a morning hug to start the day with positivity or an evening embrace to unwind, create rituals that anchor the therapeutic power of hugs into your daily schedule. These rituals serve as anchors, reminding you to prioritize emotional connection and self-care amidst the hustle of daily life.

4. Solo Hugging for Self-Comfort: Embrace the notion of self-hugging as a form of self-compassion. In moments of stress or self-doubt, wrap your arms around yourself in a comforting gesture. This self-hugging practice taps into the neurological benefits of touch, providing a tangible expression of self-love and reassurance during challenging times.

5. Bringing Hugs to the Workplace: Challenge the norm by introducing a culture of embracing in the workplace. Start team meetings with a brief moment of connection, allowing colleagues to exchange supportive hugs. This intentional practice fosters a sense

of unity, reduces workplace tension, and enhances overall morale. The workplace becomes a space where emotional well-being is prioritized alongside professional success.

6. Hugging Meditation: Explore the practice of hugging meditation as a form of mindfulness. Whether alone or with a partner, engage in a slow and intentional hug. Focus on the sensations, the rhythm of breath, and the connection formed. This meditative approach to hugging enhances self-awareness, promotes relaxation, and deepens the therapeutic impact of the embrace.

In embracing the practical insights outlined in this chapter, readers are equipped with a toolbox of techniques to seamlessly incorporate therapeutic hugs into their daily lives. From cultivating a culture of embracing in relationships to solo hugging for self-comfort, these actionable strategies empower individuals to harness the profound potential of hugs as a daily practice for emotional well-being.

The Therapeutic Hug Across Relationships:

As we conclude the chapter, we broaden our perspective to explore how therapeutic hugs can enhance various relationships. From family dynamics to friendships and romantic connections, readers will discover how the intentional practice of therapeutic hugging can deepen bonds and contribute to the overall emotional health of individuals and communities.

The therapeutic hug, with its profound ability to heal and nurture emotional well-being, extends its reach across the diverse landscapes of relationships. This exploration delves into the unique dynamics of therapeutic hugging within various relationship contexts, shedding light on how this simple yet potent act becomes a cornerstone for connection, understanding, and resilience.

1. Romantic Relationships: In the realm of romantic connections, the therapeutic hug takes on an intimate significance. Beyond

physical closeness, a warm and meaningful embrace becomes a silent language of reassurance and support. Through the ebb and flow of emotions, partners discover that the therapeutic hug serves as a powerful tool to strengthen the emotional bonds that underpin a healthy and thriving relationship. It becomes a refuge where love and vulnerability intertwine, fostering a deep sense of connection.

2. Familial Bonds: Within the tapestry of family dynamics, the therapeutic hug assumes a role of profound significance. From parent-child embraces to sibling hugs, the act becomes a thread that weaves a sense of security and belonging. Therapeutic hugging in families creates a foundation of emotional support, nurturing a space where members can find solace, express love, and navigate the complexities of familial relationships with resilience.

3. Friendships: Among friends, the therapeutic hug transcends the boundaries of

platonic connection. It becomes a gesture that communicates empathy, understanding, and solidarity. Whether celebrating shared victories or consoling during challenging times, friends discover that the therapeutic hug is a universal language that strengthens the bonds of friendship, fostering a sense of camaraderie that withstands the tests of time.

4. Professional Relationships: In the professional sphere, the therapeutic hug emerges as a unique yet impactful tool for cultivating a positive and supportive work environment. Colleagues engaging in a brief hug before meetings or during moments of stress find that this act creates a shared understanding and camaraderie. The workplace becomes a space where the therapeutic hug contributes to improved collaboration, reduced tension, and an enhanced sense of well-being among team members.

5. Mentorship and Guidance: Within mentorship dynamics, the therapeutic hug

becomes a symbol of encouragement and guidance. Mentors and mentees often find that this physical expression of support transcends professional realms, creating an emotional connection that fortifies the mentorship relationship. The therapeutic hug becomes a testament to shared growth, mutual respect, and a bond that extends beyond the professional sphere.

In navigating the diverse landscapes of relationships, the therapeutic hug emerges as a versatile and universal language. It speaks to the core of human connection, fostering understanding, resilience, and a shared journey through life's highs and lows. Regardless of the relationship context, the therapeutic hug remains a timeless and invaluable tool, reminding us that in the embrace of another, we find not only comfort but a profound affirmation of our shared humanity.

The intentional practice of therapeutic hugging goes beyond a spontaneous expression of affection; it becomes a deliberate and conscious effort to foster emotional connections, strengthen bonds, and contribute to the overall well-being of individuals and communities. Through this intentional practice, a myriad of positive effects unfolds, weaving a tapestry of emotional health that extends its threads across various aspects of human interaction.

1. Building Trust and Connection: Intentional therapeutic hugging serves as a potent tool for building trust and deepening connections. When individuals consciously engage in the act of embracing, they communicate a willingness to be vulnerable and create a space where others feel safe to do the same. This intentional vulnerability fosters a sense of trust, laying the foundation for genuine and authentic relationships.

2. Enhancing Emotional Resilience: The intentional practice of therapeutic hugging contributes to emotional resilience on an individual and communal level. Regular,

deliberate embraces stimulate the release of oxytocin, the "love hormone," which plays a crucial role in regulating stress and promoting a sense of security. As communities adopt this intentional practice, they become better equipped to face collective challenges with a strengthened and united spirit.

3. Fostering a Culture of Empathy: Communities that intentionally embrace therapeutic hugging cultivate a culture of empathy. The act of hugging is a non-verbal expression of understanding and support, allowing individuals to connect with the emotions of others on a profound level. This intentional empathy contributes to a more compassionate and understanding community, where individuals are attuned to the needs and emotions of those around them.

4. Creating Emotional Safety Nets: Intentional therapeutic hugging creates emotional safety nets within communities. Knowing that there is a shared practice of offering and receiving support through hugs

builds a sense of security. This safety net becomes especially crucial during times of crisis or upheaval, where intentional hugs provide a tangible and immediate source of comfort, reminding individuals that they are not alone in facing adversity.

5. Strengthening Social Bonds: As individuals and communities intentionally embrace therapeutic hugging, social bonds are strengthened. The act becomes a shared experience that transcends differences and fosters a sense of unity. Whether in families, friend circles, or larger community settings, intentional hugging becomes a symbol of collective care and solidarity, reinforcing the interconnectedness of individuals within the larger social fabric.

6. Promoting Mental and Emotional Well-Being: The intentional practice of therapeutic hugging contributes significantly to the mental and emotional well-being of individuals. Regular and deliberate embraces create a positive feedback loop, where the

release of endorphins and reduction of stress hormones contribute to a more balanced and resilient emotional state. Communities that embrace this intentional practice collectively contribute to the mental health of their members.

In essence, the intentional practice of therapeutic hugging emerges as a transformative force that transcends individual experiences, reaching into the collective emotional health of communities. By weaving intentional hugs into the fabric of daily interactions, individuals and communities create a resilient and compassionate foundation that fosters genuine connections, promotes empathy, and contributes to the overall emotional well-being of all involved.

In "Hug Me Close: The Art of Hugging," Chapter 3 invites readers to embrace not just for the sake of affection but as a deliberate act of self-care and emotional healing. Through the therapeutic power of hugs, we uncover a path to a more resilient and emotionally fulfilling life.

CHAPTER FOUR

The Art of Giving and Receiving Hugs

As we continue our exploration of "Hug Me Close: The Art of Hugging," Chapter 4 beckons us to delve into the intricate dance of giving and receiving hugs. In this chapter, we unravel the nuances of this art form, understanding that the exchange of embraces is a profound interaction that goes beyond the surface.

Reading Cues and Signals:

The art of giving and receiving hugs begins with the ability to read cues and signals. This section explores the unspoken language that precedes a hug – the subtle shifts in body language, the glint in the eyes, and the emotional atmosphere. Readers will gain insights into recognizing when a hug is needed, wanted, or perhaps when it's best to offer a more subtle form of support.

Hugging is a profound form of human connection, a gesture that transcends words and speaks directly to the heart. However, the true art of hugging lies not just in the embrace itself, but in the ability to read the subtle cues and signals that precede it.

1. Body Language:

The body communicates a language of its own, often expressing emotions that words fail to convey. A person in need of a hug may exhibit subtle signs such as slumped shoulders, a downturned gaze, or closed-off posture. Conversely, open body language, leaning in, or a gentle touch on their own arm may signal a desire for connection. Observing these nuances helps us discern the unspoken need for comfort.

2. The Glint in the Eyes:

Eyes are windows to the soul, revealing emotions that words may conceal. A longing, vulnerability, or a hint of sadness may manifest in the eyes, signaling a silent plea for reassurance. Equally, a sparkle of joy, excitement, or gratitude can signify a moment worthy of celebration through a warm embrace. Paying attention to these visual cues deepens our understanding of the emotional landscape.

3. Emotional Atmosphere:

The atmosphere surrounding an individual is charged with energy, and emotional currents are often palpable. Tension, sorrow, or fatigue may linger in the air, creating an opportunity for a comforting hug. Conversely, moments of shared happiness, accomplishment, or relief can invite a joyous embrace. Sensing the emotional climate allows us to respond with empathy and support when it is needed most.

4. Recognizing the Need for Space:

While hugs are a powerful means of connection, not everyone may feel comfortable receiving them at all times. Reading cues also involves recognizing when a person may need space or prefers a different form of support. Respect for personal boundaries ensures that our gestures are welcomed and appreciated.

In mastering the art of hugging, we learn to navigate the delicate dance of human connection with grace and sensitivity. By attentively interpreting the cues and signals, we can offer comfort and support in the most profound and unspoken ways. After all, the magic of a hug lies not just in the physical embrace but in the genuine understanding that precedes it.

Understanding Personal Boundaries:

Central to the art of hugging is the understanding of personal boundaries. We navigate the delicate balance between expressing warmth and respecting individual comfort zones. Through anecdotes and practical tips, readers will learn how to approach hugs with sensitivity, ensuring that each embrace is a consensual and mutually enjoyable experience.

In the realm of heartfelt embraces, a crucial element lies in the delicate dance of understanding and respecting personal boundaries. As we seek to express warmth through hugs, it becomes imperative to recognize and honor the individual comfort zones of those around us. This section delves into anecdotes and practical tips, providing readers with insights on approaching hugs with sensitivity for a consensual and mutually enjoyable experience.

1. The Uniqueness of Personal Space:

Each person's comfort zone is as unique as their fingerprint. Some individuals find solace in tight, prolonged hugs, while others may prefer a brief and gentle touch. Acknowledging the diversity of personal space preferences is the first step in fostering a culture of respectful connection.

2. Consent as a Foundation:

Consent is the cornerstone of any meaningful interaction, and hugging is no exception. Before offering or receiving a hug, it's essential to gauge the other person's willingness. Non-verbal cues, such as open body language or a welcoming smile, often signal consent. However, verbal communication may be necessary, especially in new or unfamiliar relationships.

3. Mutual Comfort as the Goal:

A successful hug is one where both parties feel comfortable and supported. Pay attention to the other person's response during the embrace. If you sense any signs of discomfort, be prepared to adjust the intensity or duration of the hug accordingly. Creating an environment where both individuals feel at ease contributes to the positive impact of the gesture.

4. Tailoring Hugs to Relationships:

Different relationships warrant varying degrees of intimacy. While close friends or family members may appreciate more extended and heartfelt hugs, acquaintances or colleagues may prefer a lighter touch. Understanding the nature of your relationship with someone helps tailor your embrace to their comfort level.

5. Offering Alternatives:

Not everyone may be receptive to hugs, and that's perfectly acceptable. Be attuned to cues indicating a preference for alternative forms of support, such as a friendly handshake, a pat on the back, or even a verbal expression of empathy. Respecting these preferences ensures that your intention to provide comfort is communicated in a way that aligns with the other person's comfort zone.

In the art of hugging, the understanding of personal boundaries transforms each embrace into a respectful and enriching experience. By navigating the fine balance between warmth and respect, we create a space where the power of human connection can be celebrated without compromising individual comfort.

The Varieties of Hug Styles:

This section delves into the diverse array of hug styles and how they cater to different needs and contexts. From the quick and casual greeting hug to the more lingering and intimate embrace, readers will explore how adapting one's hug style can enhance the quality of the interaction. The chapter emphasizes the importance of matching the right hug to the right moment.

Hugging is an art that transcends uniformity, offering a rich tapestry of styles that cater to diverse needs and contexts. This section invites readers to explore the nuanced world of hug styles, understanding how each embraces a unique purpose, and how adapting one's approach can elevate the quality of human interactions. From the brisk and casual greeting hug to the lingering and intimate embrace, this chapter underscores the significance of matching the right hug to the right moment.

1. The Casual Greeting Hug:

This quick and light embrace serves as a friendly introduction or a familiar greeting. It is often characterized by a brief touch, conveying warmth and connection without delving into deep emotional intimacy. Ideal for acquaintances, colleagues, or casual social encounters, the casual greeting hug sets a positive tone without overwhelming the interaction.

2. The Comforting Embrace:

In moments of distress or sadness, the comforting embrace offers solace and support. This style involves a longer and more enveloping hug, providing a sense of security and reassurance. It communicates empathy and a willingness to share in the other person's emotions, fostering a deeper connection during times of vulnerability.

3. The Celebratory Hug:

Shared joy and triumph are beautifully encapsulated in the celebratory hug. Characterized by enthusiasm and often accompanied by a slight lift or spin, this style radiates positivity and camaraderie. Whether it's a personal achievement, a special occasion, or a reunion, the celebratory hug amplifies the elation of the moment.

4. The Intimate Embrace:

Reserved for close relationships, the intimate embrace is a profound expression of love, affection, and connection. It involves a longer duration, a tighter hold, and often includes elements of physical closeness, such as hand-holding. This hug style deepens emotional bonds and signifies a level of trust that goes beyond mere formality.

5. The Professional Hug:

In the workplace or formal settings, a more reserved and controlled hug style is appropriate. The professional hug maintains a balance between warmth and professionalism, avoiding excessive physical contact. This style is suitable for expressing support, congratulating achievements, or consoling without compromising the boundaries of a professional relationship.

Matching the Right Hug to the Right Moment:

Understanding the nuances of each hug style empowers individuals to adapt their approach based on the specific needs and dynamics of a situation. Whether it's a casual encounter, a moment of shared joy, or a time of emotional vulnerability, choosing the appropriate hug style enhances the overall quality of human connections. In the world of hugs, versatility becomes the key to fostering meaningful and authentic relationships.

Expressing Authenticity in Hugs:

At the heart of the art lies authenticity. Readers will discover how genuine intentionality transforms hugs from mere gestures into meaningful connections. This section encourages individuals to approach hugging with sincerity, allowing each embrace to convey a true expression of care and affection.

In the tapestry of human connections, authenticity is the thread that weaves meaningful bonds. Within the realm of hugs, this section delves into the transformative power of genuine intentionality, elevating embraces from mere gestures to profound connections. Readers are invited to explore the essence of authenticity, understanding how sincerity can turn each hug into a true expression of care and affection.

1. The Power of Presence:

Authenticity in hugs begins with being fully present in the moment. Whether offering or receiving an embrace, focus on the person before you. Clear your mind of distractions, engage in active listening, and let the sincerity of your connection shine through. A hug, when accompanied by genuine presence, becomes a shared experience that transcends the physical realm.

2. Mindful Engagement:

Before initiating a hug, take a moment to gauge the emotional atmosphere and the other person's comfort level. Mindful engagement ensures that your intention aligns with the needs of the moment, fostering a connection built on mutual understanding and respect. Authenticity in hugs is not just about the act but about being attuned to the nuances of the shared experience.

3. Embracing Vulnerability:

True authenticity involves a willingness to embrace vulnerability. When offering a comforting hug, acknowledge and honor the other person's emotions without judgment. Allow vulnerability to be a bridge that deepens the connection, creating a safe space for both parties to express and share genuine feelings.

4. Heartfelt Communication:

Authentic hugs transcend the physical and become a form of heartfelt communication. Let your actions speak volumes, conveying emotions that words may struggle to articulate. A hug infused with authenticity is a silent dialogue, expressing care, understanding, and love in a language understood by the heart.

5. Consistency in Expression:

Cultivating authenticity in hugs requires consistency. Let your actions align with your true intentions consistently over time. Authentic connections are built on trust, and the reliability of your expressions through hugs fosters a sense of security and comfort within relationships.

6. Respecting Boundaries with Authenticity:

Even in the embrace of authenticity, respect for personal boundaries remains paramount. Authenticity in hugs is not about imposing one's own comfort level but about finding a harmonious balance that honors the needs and boundaries of both individuals involved.

In the world of hugs, authenticity is the magic that transforms a simple gesture into a profound expression of connection. By approaching each embrace with sincerity, individuals can create a tapestry of authentic relationships that stand the test of time.

Navigating Cultural and Contextual Differences:

The art of giving and receiving hugs extends across cultures, each with its own set of norms and expectations. This part of the chapter provides guidance on navigating cultural and contextual differences, ensuring that the intent behind a hug is universally understood while respecting diverse practices around the world.

In the universal language of hugs, understanding and respecting cultural and contextual differences become essential to ensure that this heartfelt expression transcends borders. This section of the chapter offers guidance on navigating the diverse landscape of hugging norms across cultures. By embracing sensitivity and awareness, individuals can bridge worlds, fostering connections that honor the rich tapestry of global diversity.

1. Research and Learn:

Before engaging in hugs across different cultures, take the time to research and learn about specific customs and expectations. What may be considered a warm and friendly gesture in one culture could be perceived differently in another. Understanding the nuances helps in approaching hugs with cultural sensitivity.

2. Observe and Adapt:

Cultural norms vary not only between countries but also within diverse communities. Observe and adapt your hugging style based on the context. Some cultures may be more reserved and prefer subtle gestures, while others embrace more openly. Pay attention to the cues and signals within the specific cultural or social setting.

3. Be Mindful of Personal Space:

Different cultures have varying concepts of personal space. While some cultures may appreciate close physical proximity during hugs, others may prefer a more reserved approach. Be mindful of the personal space boundaries of individuals from different cultural backgrounds, ensuring that your gestures are respectful and comfortable for everyone involved.

4. Non-Verbal Cues Matter:

In many cultures, non-verbal cues play a significant role in communication. Pay attention to subtle signals, such as body language and facial expressions, to gauge whether a hug is appropriate in a particular situation. A warm smile or open posture can often indicate receptiveness to a hug, while signs of discomfort should be respected.

5. Offer Alternatives:

Recognize that not all cultures are accustomed to hugging as a form of greeting or expression. Be prepared to offer alternative gestures, such as a nod, a handshake, or a respectful bow, depending on the cultural context. Respectfully acknowledging and adapting to local customs demonstrates cultural awareness and fosters positive interactions.

6. Respectful Inquiries:

When in doubt, consider respectfully inquiring about the cultural preferences regarding physical greetings. People from different backgrounds may appreciate your interest in understanding their customs, and this open dialogue can help establish a shared understanding of appropriate gestures.

Navigating cultural and contextual differences in hugging is a journey of cultural sensitivity and respect. By approaching the art of hugging with awareness and an open mind, individuals can bridge cultural gaps, fostering connections that celebrate the rich diversity of our global community.

The Impact of Body Language:

Hugs are a form of non-verbal communication, and this section delves into the role of body language in enhancing the art. Readers will explore how subtle shifts in posture, the strength of the embrace, and the duration of the hug can communicate nuanced messages. By mastering the language of body cues, individuals can elevate their hugging skills to a more profound level.

Hugs, as a form of non-verbal communication, derive their power not just from the physical touch but from the intricate language of body cues. In this section, readers will embark on a journey to understand the profound impact of body language in enhancing the art of hugging. By exploring the nuances of posture, the strength of the embrace, and the duration of the hug, individuals can master the unspoken language that elevates simple gestures to a more profound and meaningful level.

1. Posture Speaks Volumes:

The way we hold ourselves before, during, and after a hug communicates volumes. A warm and open posture signals receptivity and a genuine desire for connection. Conversely, closed-off body language may indicate hesitancy or discomfort. Mastering the art of hugging involves not only interpreting but also consciously adopting a posture that conveys authenticity and warmth.

2. The Strength of the Embrace:

The intensity of an embrace holds a wealth of emotional information. A gentle and tender hug may convey empathy, comfort, or support, while a firmer embrace can signify enthusiasm, celebration, or a deep bond of affection. Understanding the emotional nuances associated with the strength of the hug allows individuals to tailor their gestures to the specific needs of the moment.

3. Duration as an Emotional Barometer:

The duration of a hug serves as an emotional barometer, reflecting the depth of connection between individuals. A brief hug can express a quick greeting or acknowledgment, while a more prolonged embrace may signal a need for comfort or a desire to linger in a moment of shared joy. By intuitively gauging the emotional context, individuals can modulate the duration of their hugs to convey the appropriate level of support.

4. Reciprocity and Synchronization:

Successful hugging is a dance of reciprocity and synchronization. Pay attention to the other person's cues and synchronize your movements accordingly. Mirroring their body language creates a harmonious exchange, enhancing the connection and ensuring that the hug is a shared and mutually enriching experience.

5. Consistency in Non-Verbal Cues:

The impact of body language is magnified when it aligns consistently with verbal communication. A congruence between words and non-verbal cues deepens the authenticity of the interaction. Consistency in expressing emotions through both channels ensures that the message is clear, genuine, and resonates on a profound level.

By delving into the impact of body language in hugging, individuals can refine their ability to read and convey emotions through non-verbal cues. The art of hugging, when enriched by a mastery of body language, transforms each embrace into a beautifully nuanced expression of connection and understanding.

Creating Meaningful Connections:

As the chapter draws to a close, the focus turns to the ultimate goal of the art of giving and receiving hugs – creating meaningful connections. Through stories and examples, readers will witness the transformative power of a well-timed hug in building trust, strengthening bonds, and fostering a sense of belonging. The art of hugging becomes a pathway to enriching the tapestry of human connections.

As we conclude this chapter, we shift our focus to the ultimate goal that underpins the art of giving and receiving hugs – the creation of meaningful connections. Through stories and examples, readers will witness the transformative power of a well-timed hug in building trust, strengthening bonds, and fostering a profound sense of belonging. The art of hugging becomes a sacred pathway to enriching the vibrant tapestry of human connections.

1. Building Trust through Vulnerability:

A well-executed hug has the ability to break down walls and build trust through shared vulnerability. The vulnerability of opening oneself to an embrace fosters an environment where authenticity flourishes. Stories of individuals trusting each other enough to share a comforting hug during challenging times exemplify the role of vulnerability in forging deep, meaningful connections.

2. Strengthening Bonds in Shared Joy:

The art of hugging is not only a comfort in times of need but a celebration in moments of joy. The shared elation expressed through celebratory hugs strengthens bonds, creating lasting memories and deepening connections. Tales of friends embracing after significant achievements or families coming together in jubilant reunions illustrate the power of hugs in weaving the fabric of shared happiness.

3. Fostering Belonging and Inclusion:

Hugs have the remarkable ability to foster a sense of belonging and inclusion. Thoughtful and inclusive hugs transcend boundaries, welcoming individuals into a community of care and understanding. Stories of diverse groups embracing one another, transcending differences through shared expressions of warmth, showcase how the art of hugging can contribute to building a more compassionate and united world.

4. A Universal Language of Compassion:

The beauty of hugs lies in their universality as a language of compassion. Regardless of cultural or linguistic differences, the warmth of a hug communicates a shared humanity. Narratives of individuals from various backgrounds finding solace and connection through the simple act of hugging exemplify how this universal language transcends barriers, creating bridges between hearts.

5. Enriching the Tapestry of Human Connections:

In weaving together the stories and examples of meaningful connections forged through the art of hugging, we see the tapestry of human connections being enriched and expanded. Each embrace contributes to the intricate patterns of understanding, empathy, and love that bind us together as a global community.

The art of hugging, when practiced with intention and authenticity, becomes a powerful force for creating a world where meaningful connections flourish.

As we close this chapter, may the lessons and stories shared inspire a deeper appreciation for the art of hugging as a transformative and universal means of creating connections that resonate with the shared essence of our shared humanity.

In "Hug Me Close: The Art of Hugging," Chapter 4 invites readers to embrace the artistry inherent in every hug. By honing the skills of reading cues, respecting boundaries, and expressing authenticity, individuals can elevate their hugging experiences, creating moments of connection that resonate far beyond the physical embrace.

CHAPTER FIVE
Hugs Across Generations

In the heart-warming tapestry of "Hug Me Close: The Art of Hugging," Chapter 5 invites readers to embark on a journey that transcends time and age. Here, we celebrate the universal appeal of hugs, recognizing them as a language that seamlessly bridges the generation gap, fostering connections that endure through the ages.

The Tender Embrace of Parental Love:

Our exploration begins with the timeless embrace shared between parents and their children. This section delves into the profound significance of parental hugs, exploring how the warmth of a mother's or father's embrace provides a foundation of love and security. Readers will witness the enduring power of these embraces to shape a child's emotional landscape and contribute to their sense of well-being.

In the vast tapestry of human connections, none is more profound than the tender embrace shared between parents and their children. This section embarks on an exploration of the timeless significance of parental hugs, uncovering the inherent warmth that radiates from a mother's or father's embrace. Through stories and reflections, readers will witness the enduring power of these embraces to shape a child's emotional landscape, providing a foundation of love and security that contributes immeasurably to their sense of well-being.

1. The Cradle of Unconditional Love:

Parental hugs form the cradle of unconditional love, a sanctuary where children find solace and acceptance. The gentle, reassuring arms of a mother or father create an emotional haven, fostering an environment where a child feels cherished and valued. These hugs become the cornerstone of a bond that transcends time, offering a sense of security that accompanies the child throughout their journey into adulthood.

2. Shaping Emotional Resilience:

The power of parental hugs extends beyond the physical embrace, playing a pivotal role in shaping a child's emotional resilience. In times of sorrow, disappointment, or uncertainty, a parent's hug becomes a refuge – a silent affirmation that they are not alone. These embraces instill a deep-seated belief in the child's ability to navigate life's challenges with the unwavering support of their parents.

3. A Language of Comfort and Reassurance:

Parental hugs speak a language of comfort and reassurance that surpasses words. Whether in moments of triumph or during setbacks, the embrace communicates a profound message of love and belief in the child's potential. These gestures become an unspoken dialogue, strengthening the emotional connection between parent and child.

4. Building Trust and Security:

Through consistent and affectionate hugs, parents build a foundation of trust and security in their child's world. The physical closeness fosters a sense of safety that allows the child to explore and discover the world, knowing that a loving embrace awaits them upon their return. This trust becomes the bedrock for the child's healthy emotional development.

5. Lasting Impacts on Well-being:

The enduring impacts of parental hugs on a child's well-being are immeasurable. Research suggests that children who receive affectionate physical touch and embraces tend to develop better emotional regulation, empathy, and mental well-being. The legacy of these hugs echoes throughout a child's life, influencing their relationships, self-esteem, and overall happiness.

As we delve into the tender embrace of parental love, let us appreciate the profound role these hugs play in shaping the emotional landscape of a child. In the arms of their parents, children find not just physical warmth but the nurturing embrace that forms the cornerstone of a lifetime of love and security.

The Bond Between Siblings:

Moving through the familial spectrum, we explore the unique dynamics of sibling hugs. From the playful embraces of childhood to the supportive hugs in adulthood, readers will gain insights into how sibling hugs play a pivotal role in shaping lifelong bonds. This section illuminates the resilience and comfort that sibling embraces offer, fostering connections that evolve and adapt across the years.

As we navigate the intricate tapestry of familial relationships, the spotlight now turns to the unique dynamics of sibling hugs. This section unveils the multifaceted nature of sibling embraces, capturing the essence of playful hugs in childhood and the supportive embraces that endure into adulthood. Readers will gain insights into how these hugs play a pivotal role in shaping lifelong bonds, highlighting the resilience and comfort they offer while fostering connections that evolve and adapt across the years.

1. Playful Embraces of Childhood:

The early years of siblinghood are marked by a symphony of playful embraces. From laughter-filled hugs after shared adventures to comforting embraces during challenging times, siblings forge a unique bond through their physical expressions of affection. These childhood hugs become the threads that weave the fabric of shared memories and shared growth.

2. Supportive Hugs in Adulthood:

As siblings journey through life, the nature of their hugs evolves, transitioning from playful to supportive. In adulthood, hugs become a source of comfort, reassurance, and solidarity during life's triumphs and tribulations. Siblings stand as pillars of support, their embraces conveying an unspoken understanding that comes from a shared history and a familial connection that endures.

3. Shared Milestones and Celebrations:

Sibling hugs often punctuate shared milestones and celebrations, creating a tapestry of joy and camaraderie. From graduations and weddings to the arrival of new family members, these embraces become markers of shared happiness and a testament to the enduring nature of sibling connections. Each hug carries the weight of shared experiences and a deep-rooted bond that transcends time.

4. Weathering Storms Together:

Life's storms are inevitable, and it is during these turbulent times that sibling hugs gain a profound significance. Whether it's the loss of a loved one, personal struggles, or challenging transitions, the embrace of a sibling serves as a constant amidst uncertainty. The shared resilience in facing adversity strengthens the bond, creating a support system that stands firm in the face of life's challenges.

5. Evolving Connections Across Years:

The beauty of sibling hugs lies in their ability to adapt and evolve across the years. From the spontaneous hugs of childhood to the intentional embraces of adulthood, siblings navigate the complexities of life together. The hugs become a language of their own, speaking to the enduring connection that withstands the test of time.

As we explore the bond between siblings through the lens of hugs, we discover a profound narrative of shared experiences, resilience, and unwavering support. Through playful embraces in youth to the supportive hugs in later years, siblings craft a unique connection that enriches the journey of life, weaving a tapestry of love and shared memories that endure across the ages.

Friends Forever: The Enthusiastic Hug of Friendship:

This part of the chapter focuses on the exuberant hugs exchanged between friends. Regardless of age, friends share a unique bond that often finds expression in embraces filled with laughter, understanding, and shared experiences. Through stories and anecdotes, readers will witness the joyous celebration of friendship through the language of hugs, illustrating the timeless nature of camaraderie.

In the vibrant mosaic of human connections, the spotlight now turns to the exuberant hugs exchanged between friends. This section of the chapter dives into the enthusiastic and joyful embraces that define the unique bond of friendship. Regardless of age, friends share a connection that finds expression in hugs filled with laughter, understanding, and the warmth of shared experiences. Through stories and anecdotes, readers will embark on a journey to witness the joyous celebration of friendship through the language of hugs, illustrating the timeless nature of camaraderie.

1. The Laughter-Filled Embrace:

Friendship hugs are often characterized by unbridled enthusiasm and infectious laughter. Whether it's a reunion after a long time apart or a spontaneous celebration of shared victories, friends greet each other with hugs that radiate pure joy. These laughter-filled embraces become a language of their own, expressing the delight of being in the company of kindred spirits.

2. Understanding in Silence:

Friends share a unique ability to understand each other without the need for words. The enthusiastic hug of friendship goes beyond verbal communication, embodying an unspoken understanding and acceptance. Whether in times of triumph or moments of vulnerability, the embrace becomes a silent affirmation of support and companionship.

3. Celebrating Shared Experiences:

Friendship hugs are a celebration of shared experiences, marking the highs and lows of life's journey. From the adventures that create lasting memories to the challenges that strengthen the bond, friends express their connection through embraces that encapsulate the richness of their shared history.

4. Timeless Camaraderie:

The nature of friendship hugs transcends the passage of time. Regardless of how many years have elapsed since the last meeting, friends have a remarkable ability to pick up where they left off. The enthusiastic hug serves as a timeless reminder of the enduring camaraderie that withstands the tests of distance and change.

5. The Comfort of Companionship:

In the enthusiastic hug of friendship, there is a comforting reassurance that one is not alone on life's journey. Friends provide a support system that brings solace in times of need and amplifies the joy in moments of celebration.

The embrace becomes a refuge, a tangible expression of the comfort found in the company of true friends.

As we delve into the world of friendship hugs, filled with laughter, understanding, and shared experiences, we witness the timeless nature of camaraderie. Through the language of hugs, friends express the joy of companionship, creating a mosaic of warmth and connection that stands as a testament to the enduring power of true friendship.

Generational Bridging Through Hugs:

As we delve deeper, this section explores the unique role hugs play in bridging generational gaps. From grandparents showering affection on their grandchildren to the reciprocal support exchanged between different age groups, readers will gain a profound understanding of how hugs become a medium through which generations connect, share wisdom, and pass on the warmth of familial traditions.

In the rich tapestry of human relationships, the section now unravels the unique role hugs play in bridging generational gaps. From grandparents showering affection on their grandchildren to the reciprocal support exchanged between different age groups, readers will gain a profound understanding of how hugs become a medium through which generations connect, share wisdom, and pass on the warmth of familial traditions.

1. Grandparental Affection:

The embrace shared between grandparents and grandchildren is a tender dance of affection that transcends time. Grandparents, with a lifetime of experiences etched on their hearts, use hugs to impart love, wisdom, and a sense of familial continuity. In the warmth of their arms, grandchildren find a connection to the past and a bridge to the future.

2. Passing Down Traditions:

Hugs become a medium through which traditions are passed down from one generation to the next. Whether it's the warmth of a familial embrace during holidays, the embrace of shared values, or the passing on of cultural practices, hugs carry the weight of heritage. Through these gestures, older generations sow the seeds of tradition, ensuring that the essence of family is preserved and celebrated.

3. The Reciprocal Exchange:

Generational bridging through hugs is not a one-way street; it is a reciprocal exchange that enriches both the givers and receivers. The older generation imparts wisdom and love, while the younger generation provides a fresh perspective and vitality. Hugs become a symbol of mutual respect and understanding, fostering an intergenerational connection that is both dynamic and enduring.

4. Supportive Embraces:

In times of challenge or change, hugs act as a source of support between different age groups. Whether it's a comforting embrace from a parent to a child navigating the complexities of adolescence or the reassuring hug from a grown child to an aging parent, these gestures become a lifeline of comfort and strength.

5. Shared Milestones and Celebrations:

Generational hugs punctuate shared milestones and celebrations, creating a continuum of familial joy and accomplishment. From the exuberant hug of grandparents witnessing the achievements of their grandchildren to the heartfelt embraces exchanged during family gatherings, these moments become snapshots of shared happiness that bridge the gaps between generations.

6. A Tapestry of Connection:

In the embrace of different age groups, a tapestry of connection is woven. Each hug contributes a thread to the intricate fabric of family bonds, creating a resilient and beautiful mosaic that withstands the passage of time. Generational bridging through hugs encapsulates the essence of continuity, love, and the interwoven stories that shape the family narrative.

As we explore the role of hugs in bridging generational gaps, we witness a timeless thread that connects the past, present, and future. Through these gestures, generations intertwine, sharing not only embraces but also the invaluable gifts of love, wisdom, and the enduring legacy of familial connections.

Intergenerational Hugging Traditions:

Within families and communities, hugging often becomes a cherished tradition passed down through generations. This part of the chapter delves into the continuity of hugging practices, examining how specific embraces become symbols of familial ties, linking ancestors with descendants. Through this exploration, readers will come to appreciate the role of hugs in weaving a tapestry of continuity and connection.

Within the fabric of families and communities, hugging often transcends the ordinary to become a cherished tradition passed down through generations. This segment of the chapter delves into the continuity of hugging practices, exploring how specific embraces evolve into symbols of familial ties, seamlessly linking ancestors with descendants. Through this exploration, readers will come to appreciate the profound role of hugs in weaving a tapestry of continuity and connection that spans across time.

1. Rituals of Affection:

Intergenerational hugging traditions often manifest as rituals of affection, where specific embraces are woven into the fabric of family life. From the bear hugs passed down from grandparents to parents and then to children, to the gentle embraces shared between siblings and cousins, these rituals serve as a timeless expression of familial love that withstands the test of time.

2. Symbolic Gestures:

Certain hugs within a family become symbolic gestures, representing more than just physical affection. These embraces carry the weight of shared values, cultural heritage, and the enduring bonds that tie generations together. They become a language of their own, conveying a legacy of love that stretches across the ages.

3. Passing Down Wisdom Through Hugs:

Intergenerational hugging traditions often serve as a conduit for passing down wisdom. The embrace of an elder becomes not only a gesture of love but a transfer of lessons learned, experiences gained, and insights accumulated over a lifetime. In these hugs, the younger generation finds a wellspring of knowledge, connecting them to the wealth of familial wisdom.

4. Celebratory Embraces Across Generations:

From birth to milestones like graduations, weddings, and the welcoming of new family members, celebratory embraces become a consistent thread woven through the generations. The shared joy in these embraces serves as a living testament to the continuity of familial bonds, creating a sense of unity that extends beyond individual lifetimes.

5. Adaptive Traditions:

As families evolve and adapt to changing times, hugging traditions also undergo transformations. While the essence of familial warmth remains constant, the specific expressions of affection may adapt to reflect the values and customs of each era. These adaptive traditions ensure that hugging remains a relevant and meaningful practice for each generation.

6. Creating a Legacy of Connection:

Intergenerational hugging traditions, when passed down with intention and love, create a legacy of connection. Each hug becomes a link in a chain that connects ancestors, present generations, and those yet to come.

This legacy is not only a celebration of familial ties but also a testament to the enduring power of human connection through the simple yet profound act of hugging.

In the continuum of intergenerational hugging traditions, families find a source of strength, love, and continuity. Through these cherished embraces, generations connect in a dance of affection, creating a tapestry that tells the story of familial ties that endure through time.

The Power of the Elderly Embrace:

This section highlights the significance of hugs in the lives of the elderly. Whether it's the comforting embrace of a grandparent or the support offered by an older friend, hugs play a crucial role in promoting emotional well-being in the later stages of life. Readers will witness how these embraces contribute to a sense of belonging and purpose for seniors, fostering emotional resilience and vitality.

In the later stages of life, the significance of hugs takes on a profound meaning, offering emotional sustenance and connectivity to the elderly. This section unveils the transformative power of elderly embraces, whether it's the comforting hug of a grandparent or the supportive embrace of an older friend. Readers will witness how these hugs play a crucial role in promoting emotional well-being, contributing to a sense of belonging and purpose for seniors and fostering emotional resilience and vitality.

1. Comforting Grandparental Embraces:

The embrace of a grandparent holds a unique power in the lives of both the elderly and their grandchildren. In the gentle arms of a grandparent, there's a comforting reassurance that transcends words. These hugs convey a sense of continuity, bridging generations and providing a source of love and stability that remains unwavering.

2. Supportive Embraces from Older Friends:

As individuals age, the support of friends becomes increasingly precious. The hugs exchanged between older friends hold a special significance, providing a sense of camaraderie and understanding that comes from shared experiences. These embraces become pillars of support, fostering a sense of connection that is vital for emotional well-being in the later stages of life.

3. Combatting Loneliness and Isolation:

For many seniors, the embrace becomes a powerful antidote to the loneliness and isolation that can accompany aging. Whether it's a hug from a family member, friend, or caregiver, these gestures bridge the gap created by physical distance and offer a tangible reminder of human connection, reducing feelings of solitude.

4. Fostering Emotional Resilience:

Elderly embraces contribute significantly to fostering emotional resilience. The physical touch and warmth inherent in hugs release oxytocin, a hormone associated with bonding and stress reduction. These biological responses contribute to a sense of emotional well-being, helping seniors navigate the emotional challenges that may arise in the later stages of life.

5. Creating a Sense of Belonging:

The power of elderly embraces lies in their ability to create a profound sense of belonging. In a world that may seem increasingly unfamiliar, the embrace becomes a touchstone of familiarity and love. Whether it's a familial hug or a hug exchanged with friends, this sense of belonging contributes to a positive outlook and a greater overall quality of life for seniors.

6. Vitality and Joy Through Connection:

Embraces in later life are not just about physical touch but about nurturing a connection that brings vitality and joy. The shared laughter, stories, and warmth exchanged in hugs contribute to an emotional vibrancy that enhances the overall well-being of seniors, showcasing the enduring power of human connection.

In the twilight of life, the power of elderly embraces illuminates the path to emotional well-being, offering comfort, support, and a profound sense of connection. Through these gestures, the elderly continue to enrich their lives and the lives of those around them, demonstrating that the transformative power of hugs knows no age limit.

Fostering Emotionally Connected Communities:

In the concluding part of the chapter, the focus broadens to the communal level, celebrating how intergenerational hugging fosters emotionally connected communities. By recognizing the universality of the hug across generations, readers will gain insights into how these simple acts contribute to the fabric of society, creating communities that thrive on compassion, understanding, and shared affection.

As we conclude this chapter, the lens widens to celebrate how intergenerational hugging fosters emotionally connected communities. The embrace, transcending age and backgrounds, becomes a universal language that enriches the fabric of society. Readers will gain insights into how these simple acts contribute to the tapestry of communal life, creating communities that thrive on compassion, understanding, and shared affection.

1. Breaking Down Generational Barriers:

Intergenerational hugging serves as a powerful tool in breaking down barriers between different age groups within a community. The embrace becomes a bridge that connects the wisdom of older generations with the energy and innovation of the younger ones. In these shared moments, a sense of unity and understanding flourishes, fostering a community where individuals of all ages feel valued and interconnected.

2. Fostering Empathy and Compassion:

The act of hugging, regardless of age, fosters empathy and compassion within communities. When individuals of diverse backgrounds and experiences come together in shared embraces, they build a foundation of mutual understanding. These moments of connection create a culture of empathy, enhancing the overall emotional well-being of the community.

3. Nurturing a Sense of Belonging:

In emotionally connected communities, the embrace becomes a symbol of belonging. Whether it's the familial hug exchanged between generations or the supportive embrace offered among friends and neighbors, the act of hugging reinforces the notion that each individual is an integral part of the community tapestry. This sense of belonging fosters a collective spirit that transcends individual differences.

4. Strengthening Social Bonds:

Communities enriched by intergenerational hugging witness strengthened social bonds. The shared affection contributes to a sense of unity, cooperation, and mutual support. As community members actively engage in the act of hugging, they contribute to a culture of interconnectedness that weaves together the diverse threads of their shared experiences.

5. Celebrating Diversity through Affection:

Hugs within emotionally connected communities celebrate the diversity of backgrounds, cultures, and life experiences. The act of embracing becomes a universal language that transcends differences, fostering an atmosphere of acceptance and appreciation for the rich tapestry of community life. Each hug becomes a celebration of the unique contributions individuals bring to the collective whole.

6. The Ripple Effect of Connection:

The impact of intergenerational hugging goes beyond individual exchanges; it creates a ripple effect of connection that extends throughout the community. As individuals experience the warmth and understanding inherent in these embraces, they, in turn, contribute to the creation of a more compassionate and emotionally connected community.

In the final analysis, the universal language of hugs weaves a thread of emotional connection that binds communities together. Recognizing the transformative power of these simple acts, communities can embrace a culture of compassion, understanding, and shared affection that resonates across generations, creating a harmonious and thriving collective tapestry.

In "Hug Me Close: The Art of Hugging," Chapter 5 celebrates the timeless appeal of hugs, demonstrating their ability to transcend age barriers and cultivate emotionally rich connections that endure through the tapestry of generations.

CHAPTER SIX

Navigating Cultural Hugging Etiquette

In the intricate tapestry of global connections, Chapter 6 of "Hug Me Close: The Art of Hugging" ventures into the rich landscape of cultural diversity. Here, we explore the fascinating realm of hugging etiquettes around the world, acknowledging the importance of respecting cultural nuances to truly embrace the art of hugging with sensitivity and appreciation.

The Global Language of Hugs:

As we embark on this cultural exploration, it's crucial to recognize that while hugs are a universal form of communication, their expression is deeply influenced by cultural contexts. This section emphasizes the shared human experience that hugs offer while laying the foundation for understanding the unique variations that make each cultural hugging etiquette distinct.

Embarking on a cultural exploration, it's essential to recognize hugs as a universal form of communication, a global language that transcends borders. This section emphasizes the shared human experience that hugs offer while laying the foundation for understanding the unique variations that make each cultural hugging etiquette distinct.

1. The Universality of Human Connection:

Hugs serve as a universal expression of human connection, uniting people across continents and cultures. Regardless of language or background, the act of embracing conveys a shared understanding of our fundamental need for warmth, support, and affection. It becomes a global language that speaks to the common threads of the human experience.

2. Cultural Variations in Hugging Etiquette:

While the desire for connection is universal, the expression of hugs is deeply influenced by cultural contexts. This section delves into the rich tapestry of cultural variations in hugging etiquette, recognizing that the meaning, frequency, and appropriateness of hugs can vary widely from one culture to another. Understanding these nuances is crucial in navigating diverse social landscapes.

3. Respect for Personal Space:

Cultural hugging etiquette often reflects varying norms regarding personal space. Some cultures embrace closeness and physical contact, viewing hugs as a warm and natural way to express affection. In contrast, others may prioritize personal space and reserve physical contact for more intimate relationships. Respecting these cultural differences ensures that the intent behind a hug is universally understood.

4. Non-Verbal Communication Across Cultures:

Hugs, as a form of non-verbal communication, play a significant role in cross-cultural interactions. This section explores how different cultures utilize hugs as a means of expressing emotions, building trust, and establishing connections. Non-verbal cues such as body language and facial expressions become crucial in interpreting the appropriateness and intent behind a hug.

5. Rituals and Ceremonial Hugs:

Many cultures incorporate hugs into rituals and ceremonies, adding layers of cultural significance to these embraces. From celebratory hugs during festivals to solemn embraces in mourning, this section examines how hugs become woven into the fabric of cultural practices, becoming symbols of shared values, traditions, and moments of collective importance.

6. Adapting to Globalized Spaces:

In an increasingly globalized world, individuals often find themselves in multicultural environments where diverse hugging etiquettes intersect. Navigating these spaces requires cultural sensitivity, adaptability, and a willingness to understand and appreciate the varying perspectives on physical affection. Embracing the global diversity of hugging norms contributes to fostering inclusive and harmonious interactions.

As we explore the global language of hugs, it's a celebration of shared humanity while respecting and cherishing the cultural diversity that shapes our expressions of affection. Understanding the nuances of cultural hugging etiquette allows individuals to bridge gaps, build connections, and contribute to a world where the global language of hugs becomes a harmonious symphony of shared understanding and appreciation.

Dos and Don'ts: Navigating Cultural Nuances:

Delving into the heart of cultural hugging etiquettes, readers will gain insights into the dos and don'ts of embracing in various parts of the world. From the warm and expressive embraces in Latin America to the reserved and subtle hugs in some Asian cultures, this section serves as a guide to navigating cultural nuances with respect and openness.

As we delve into the heart of cultural hugging etiquettes, it's essential to navigate the diverse landscapes with respect and openness. This section serves as a guide to the dos and don'ts of embracing in various parts of the world, recognizing the rich tapestry of cultural nuances that shape the meaning and appropriateness of hugs.

Dos:

Observe and Learn:

Do: Take the time to observe and learn about the cultural norms of the community you are in. Pay attention to how people greet each other and the level of physical contact they are comfortable with.

Follow Local Initiatives:

Do: Allow locals to take the lead in initiating hugs or determining the level of physical closeness. Following their cues helps ensure that your gestures are well-received and culturally appropriate.

Respect Personal Space:

Do: Respect personal space and be aware of cultural preferences regarding physical contact. In some cultures, people may be more comfortable with personal space, while in others, closeness is embraced.

Adjust to Formality Levels:

Do: Adjust your hugging approach based on the formality of the situation. In some cultures, hugs may be reserved for close relationships, while in others, they may be common in both personal and professional settings.

Inquire About Local Customs:

Do: Inquire politely about local customs and hugging preferences, especially if you are unsure. This shows respect for the cultural nuances and a genuine interest in understanding and adapting to local practices.

Don'ts:

Assume Universality:

Don't: Assume that hugging is universally accepted in the same way. Be mindful that cultural norms vary, and what may be a warm gesture in one culture could be perceived differently in another.

Force Physical Contact:

Don't: Force physical contact or assume that everyone is comfortable with hugs. Always be sensitive to the cues and boundaries of others, particularly in cultures where personal space is highly valued.

Neglect Gender Considerations:

Don't: Neglect gender considerations. In certain cultures, there may be specific guidelines regarding physical contact between genders. Be aware of these norms and act accordingly.

Overlook Context:

Don't: Overlook the context of the interaction. Different situations may call for varying levels of physical contact. Assess the environment and adjust your hugging behavior accordingly.

Disregard Non-Verbal Cues:

Don't: Disregard non-verbal cues. Pay attention to body language and facial expressions, as they can convey whether a hug is welcomed or if it may be making someone uncomfortable.

By embracing cultural sensitivity and adapting to the dos and don'ts of each cultural context, individuals can navigate hugging etiquettes with grace and respect. This approach fosters understanding and promotes positive interactions, contributing to a global community where diverse expressions of affection are celebrated and honored.

The European Cheek-to-Cheek Embrace:

European cultures often express affection through the cheek-to-cheek embrace, varying in the number of kisses exchanged. This part of the chapter delves into the intricacies of this practice, offering readers a deeper understanding of the European hugging etiquette and the significance of this intimate form of greeting.

In the diverse tapestry of European cultures, expressions of affection often find their form in the cheek-to-cheek embrace, a practice that varies in the number of kisses exchanged. This segment of the chapter delves into the intricacies of this intimate form of greeting, offering readers a deeper understanding of European hugging etiquette and the cultural significance embedded within this unique practice.

1. The Essence of Cheek-to-Cheek:

The cheek-to-cheek embrace, commonly known as the "air kiss" or "faire la bise," is a prevalent form of greeting across many European cultures. Rather than a traditional hug, individuals lean in to lightly touch cheeks and exchange kisses in the air. The number of kisses can vary between regions, often ranging from one to three kisses.

2. Regional Variations:

Understanding the nuances of the cheek-to-cheek embrace requires awareness of regional variations. In France, for instance, the number of kisses can differ between regions, with some areas favoring two kisses while others may lean towards three. Similar variations exist in other European countries, showcasing the richness of cultural diversity within the continent.

3. The Art of Timing:

Timing is crucial in the cheek-to-cheek embrace. The exchange of kisses occurs during the initial greeting, and misjudging the timing can lead to awkward moments. Europeans often initiate the gesture by leaning in towards the right cheek, and the number of kisses is reciprocated accordingly. Being attuned to the rhythm of the greeting ensures a smooth and culturally respectful interaction.

4. Gender and Social Considerations:

Cheek-to-cheek embraces in Europe are not strictly reserved for intimate relationships; they are also commonly exchanged in social settings. However, there are considerations based on gender and social context. In some cultures, men may greet with a firm handshake or a single kiss, while women may exchange cheek kisses. Social proximity and familiarity often dictate the level of intimacy in the cheek-to-cheek embrace.

5. The Symbolism of Connection:

Beyond its surface-level form, the cheek-to-cheek embrace holds deeper symbolism. It signifies a connection, a moment of shared warmth, and an acknowledgment of the bonds between individuals. This practice emphasizes the importance of personal relationships and the role of physical touch in conveying affection and camaraderie.

6. Navigating Cultural Sensitivity:

For those engaging in European hugging etiquette, navigating cultural sensitivity is essential. Being open to the variations in cheek-to-cheek embraces and adapting to local customs demonstrates respect for cultural diversity. Awareness of the regional differences in the number of kisses and the understanding that these customs may evolve over time contribute to smooth cross-cultural interactions.

As readers delve into the intricacies of the European cheek-to-cheek embrace, they gain not only a practical understanding of hugging etiquette but also an appreciation for the cultural nuances that shape the ways people express affection. In the embrace of cheek kisses, Europe reveals a unique and intimate language of connection that adds vibrancy to its diverse cultural mosaic.

The Warm Embrace of the Mediterranean:

Mediterranean cultures are known for their warm and expressive embraces that go beyond formalities. In this section, readers will explore the genuine and enthusiastic hugging traditions that characterize the Mediterranean region, emphasizing the communal and familial nature of their embraces.

In the sun-soaked tapestry of Mediterranean cultures, the embrace is not just a formality; it is a warm and expressive tradition that radiates genuine affection. This section invites readers to explore the heartfelt and enthusiastic hugging traditions that characterize the Mediterranean region, emphasizing the communal and familial nature of these embraces.

1. Enthusiastic Greetings:

Mediterranean cultures are renowned for their enthusiastic approach to greetings, and hugs play a central role in this ritual. Whether welcoming friends, family, or acquaintances, the embrace is a heartfelt gesture that transcends mere politeness. It serves as an immediate expression of warmth and connection, reflecting the open and inclusive nature of Mediterranean societies.

2. Familial Embraces:

Within Mediterranean families, hugs are more than gestures; they are rituals that reinforce familial bonds. From grandparents to grandchildren, and among siblings and extended relatives, the embrace is a constant thread woven into the fabric of everyday life. These familial hugs express love, support, and a deep sense of belonging.

3. Symbolism of Shared Meals:

Mediterranean cultures often intertwine the act of hugging with communal gatherings, particularly during shared meals. Family and friends embrace before and after meals, marking these occasions with warmth and conviviality. The act of hugging becomes a symbolic link between the joy of companionship and the pleasure of shared food.

4. Emotional Support in Challenges:

In times of challenges or life's uncertainties, the Mediterranean embrace takes on a special significance. Friends and family offer hugs as a form of emotional support, creating a sense of solidarity in facing life's ups and downs. These embraces are not only expressions of care but also tools for building resilience within communities.

5. Spontaneity and Expressiveness:

Mediterranean hugging traditions are characterized by spontaneity and expressiveness. It is not uncommon for individuals to initiate hugs without hesitation, embracing each other with genuine joy and exuberance. This uninhibited approach to physical affection contributes to a culture where emotional connections are celebrated and valued.

6. Rituals of Reunion:

Whether it's the return of a family member, the gathering of friends, or the reunion of loved ones after a period of separation, Mediterranean cultures mark these moments with heartfelt embraces. These rituals of reunion go beyond words, encapsulating the joy and emotional richness of coming together.

As readers immerse themselves in the warm embrace of the Mediterranean, they witness a culture where hugs are not just gestures but vibrant expressions of love, connection, and communal spirit. In the genuine and enthusiastic hugging traditions of this region, the act of embracing becomes a celebration of life's interconnectedness and the enduring strength of relationships.

Asian Respect and Reserve:

In contrast, many Asian cultures demonstrate respect and reserve in their hugging customs. The chapter explores the significance of bowing and other non-contact gestures, providing readers with insights into how individuals from these cultures express affection in a more subdued manner.

In stark contrast to the warm and expressive embraces found in some cultures, many Asian cultures navigate the landscape of affection with a distinctive blend of respect and reserve. This chapter unravels the significance of bowing and other non-contact gestures, offering readers insights into how individuals from these cultures express affection in a more subdued and nuanced manner.

1. The Art of Bowing:

Bowing is a hallmark gesture in many Asian cultures, representing a deep-rooted tradition of respect and humility. The angle and depth of the bow convey various messages, from a slight nod of acknowledgment to a more profound bow expressing reverence. In lieu of physical contact, bowing becomes a nuanced way of showing deference and affection without breaching personal space.

2. Reserved Physical Contact:

In Asian cultures, the expression of affection often leans towards reserved physical contact. Hugging, especially in public or formal settings, may be considered more intimate than preferred. Individuals from these cultures may choose alternative gestures, such as a slight touch on the arm or a gentle handshake, to convey warmth without infringing on personal boundaries.

3. Gesture of Offering:

Gift-giving serves as a significant expression of affection in many Asian cultures. The act of offering a thoughtful gift is laden with symbolism, representing care, appreciation, and a desire to strengthen the relationship. In lieu of physical embraces, these tangible expressions become meaningful tokens of affection.

4. Mindful Non-Contact Gestures:

Non-contact gestures in Asian cultures often revolve around mindfulness and intentionality. Expressions of affection may include placing one's hands together in a prayer-like position, commonly seen in cultures influenced by Buddhism. These gestures carry a spiritual resonance, emphasizing the connection between the mind, body, and the shared moment.

5. Importance of Facial Expressions:

Facial expressions play a crucial role in conveying affection in Asian cultures. A warm smile, eye contact, or a slight tilt of the head can signify genuine connection and affection. The nuanced language of the face becomes a canvas for expressing emotions without the need for physical touch.

6. Cultural Context in Expressing Emotion:

Understanding the cultural context is paramount when interpreting expressions of affection in Asian cultures. Public displays of emotion, including physical contact, may be reserved for more intimate settings. This cultural nuance underscores the importance of adapting to the local customs and appreciating the diversity in how affection is communicated.

As readers explore the realm of Asian respect and reserve, they gain a profound understanding of the intricate ways in which individuals from these cultures navigate the landscape of affection. Whether through the art of bowing, reserved physical contact, or mindful non-contact gestures, the expression of warmth in Asian cultures unfolds with grace, intentionality, and a deep respect for personal boundaries.

African Richness in Ritualistic Embraces:

African cultures boast a rich tapestry of ritualistic embraces that vary across regions. Readers will discover the diverse hugging customs that showcase the continent's vibrant traditions, from intricate handshakes to full-body embraces, each carrying its own symbolic meaning.

Within the diverse landscapes of Africa, a rich tapestry of ritualistic embraces unfolds, varying across regions and showcasing the continent's vibrant traditions. This chapter invites readers to discover the multitude of hugging customs that adorn Africa, ranging from intricate handshakes to full-body embraces, each carrying its own symbolic meaning and contributing to the continent's cultural richness.

1. Intricate Handshakes:

African hugging traditions often find expression in intricate handshakes that go beyond a mere exchange of greetings. These handshakes can involve a series of movements, finger snaps, or interlocking fingers, each element adding layers of meaning. The handshake becomes a dance of connection, conveying friendship, respect, and shared cultural identity.

2. Full-Body Embraces:

In many African cultures, full-body embraces are a common form of greeting, representing a warm and expansive expression of connection. These embraces often involve a rhythmic sway or patting on the back, emphasizing the communal nature of the greeting. The physical contact extends beyond a mere gesture, embodying a sense of unity and belonging.

3. Symbolism in Touch:

African hugging customs are imbued with symbolism, and the act of touch holds profound meaning. Whether it's a gentle touch on the shoulder, a warm embrace, or the joining of hands, these gestures communicate a sense of solidarity, trust, and shared humanity. The physical connection becomes a conduit for expressing emotions that may transcend verbal communication.

4. Cultural Variations:

The diversity of Africa is reflected in the variations of hugging customs across regions and ethnic groups. From the Masai people in East Africa to the Yoruba in West Africa, each community brings its unique flair to hugging traditions. These variations add depth to the cultural mosaic of Africa, showcasing the continent's ability to celebrate diversity within unity.

5. Rituals and Ceremonial Embraces:

Ritualistic embraces are woven into the fabric of ceremonies and celebrations across Africa. Whether it's a traditional dance, a rite of passage, or a communal gathering, hugging customs play a central role in these events. The embraces become a living expression of cultural identity and shared joy, enriching the tapestry of African traditions.

6. Connection to Ancestral Roots:

African hugging customs often carry a deep connection to ancestral roots and cultural heritage. The gestures passed down through generations serve as a link to the past, fostering a sense of continuity and identity. In embracing these customs, individuals connect not only with each other but also with the timeless traditions that define their cultural legacy.

As readers embark on the exploration of African richness in ritualistic embraces, they witness a vibrant panorama of cultural expressions. From intricate handshakes to full-body embraces, each gesture contributes to the collective identity of Africa, celebrating the continent's diversity and underscoring the universal language of connection that transcends geographical boundaries.

Navigating Cross-Cultural Interactions:

This section offers practical guidance on navigating cross-cultural interactions, fostering an environment of understanding and appreciation. Readers will learn to adapt their hugging styles with cultural sensitivity, ensuring that gestures of affection are well-received and reciprocated in a manner that respects diverse cultural practices.

In the intricate dance of cross-cultural interactions, this section serves as a practical guide, offering readers insights into adapting their hugging styles with cultural sensitivity. The aim is to foster an environment of understanding and appreciation, ensuring that gestures of affection are well-received and reciprocated in a manner that respects diverse cultural practices.

1. Cultivate Cultural Awareness:

The first step in navigating cross-cultural interactions is cultivating cultural awareness. Take the time to educate yourself about the hugging customs and cultural norms of the communities you engage with. This knowledge forms the foundation for adapting your approach and expressing affection in a manner that aligns with local practices.

2. Observe and Follow Local Initiatives:

When in a new cultural setting, observe and follow local initiatives when it comes to hugging. Let the locals take the lead in initiating physical contact, and mirror their approach to ensure that your gestures are culturally appropriate. This respectful observance of local customs fosters a sense of cultural harmony.

3. Respect Personal Space:

Respecting personal space is a universal principle, but its interpretation can vary across cultures. Some cultures may embrace physical closeness, while others prioritize personal space. Be attuned to non-verbal cues and ensure that your hugging style aligns with the level of physical contact that is culturally accepted in a given context.

4. Adapt Hugging Styles:

Adaptability is key in cross-cultural hugging. Be open to adjusting your hugging style based on the cultural nuances of the community you are interacting with. Whether it's the European cheek-to-cheek embrace, the Asian bow, or the African full-body embrace, willingness to adapt showcases cultural sensitivity and a genuine respect for diversity.

5. Inquire and Communicate:

When in doubt, inquire politely about local hugging customs. Communicate with locals to understand their preferences and express your willingness to adapt. Asking questions and seeking guidance not only demonstrates cultural respect but also opens up conversations that can bridge gaps and foster mutual understanding.

6. Gauge the Formality of the Situation:

The formality of the situation can influence the appropriateness of hugging. In more formal settings, such as business or official gatherings, it's essential to gauge the level of formality and adjust your hugging style accordingly. A more reserved approach may be suitable in professional environments, while a warmer embrace may be welcomed in informal settings.

7. Be Mindful of Gender Norms:

Consider gender norms in the cultural context you find yourself in. Some cultures may have specific guidelines regarding physical contact between genders. Being mindful of these norms ensures that your hugging gestures are respectful and aligned with local expectations.

8. Embrace Flexibility and Humility:

Approaching cross-cultural interactions with flexibility and humility is paramount. Embrace the opportunity to learn from different cultural practices and be willing to adapt. Acknowledge that cultural norms may evolve, and being open to understanding and respecting these changes contributes to positive and enriching cross-cultural exchanges.

As readers internalize the principles of navigating cross-cultural interactions, they embark on a journey of mutual respect, understanding, and appreciation. Through cultural sensitivity, individuals can bridge gaps, build connections, and contribute to a global community where diverse expressions of affection are celebrated and honored.

Celebrating Diversity, Embracing Unity:

The chapter concludes by celebrating the beauty of cultural diversity in hugging etiquettes. Through the art of understanding and respecting these differences, readers will recognize that while hugs may be expressed in various ways, the underlying essence remains the same – a universal language of connection, warmth, and shared humanity.

As the final curtain descends on this chapter, we celebrate the intricate beauty of cultural diversity in hugging etiquettes. Through the art of understanding and respecting these differences, readers embark on a journey where the kaleidoscope of global hugging customs converges into a symphony of connection, warmth, and shared humanity.

1. The Mosaic of Hugging Traditions:

Our exploration has unveiled a rich mosaic of hugging traditions, from the European cheek-to-cheek embrace to the warm embraces of the Mediterranean and the respectful gestures found in Asian cultures. Each tradition adds a unique hue to the global canvas, contributing to the vibrancy of human expression.

2. Universal Essence of Connection:

Beneath the surface of diverse hugging customs lies a universal essence – the innate human desire for connection. Whether it's through the intricate handshakes of Africa, the reserved bowing of Asia, or the exuberant hugs of the Mediterranean, individuals across the globe share the common thread of seeking warmth, understanding, and connection.

3. Bridging Differences with Understanding:

Understanding and respecting these differences become the bridge that spans cultures. By delving into the nuances of hugging etiquettes, readers have acquired the tools to navigate cross-cultural interactions with grace, ensuring that gestures of affection are met with understanding and reciprocation.

4. Embracing the Tapestry of Shared Humanity:

As readers reflect on the diverse hugging traditions explored in this chapter, they come to embrace the tapestry of shared humanity. The various forms of embraces, whether simple or intricate, become threads that weave individuals together, transcending geographical, linguistic, and cultural boundaries.

5. A Call to Celebrate:

The chapter concludes with a call to celebrate the beauty found in the diversity of hugging etiquettes. Rather than seeing differences as barriers, readers are encouraged to view them as vibrant expressions of human creativity and cultural richness. In celebrating this diversity, we affirm the importance of honoring the uniqueness that each culture brings to the collective story of humanity.

6. The Legacy of Hugging Traditions:

Hugging traditions leave behind a legacy that extends beyond the present moment. As readers engage with the cultural nuances of embracing, they contribute to a legacy of mutual respect, cross-cultural understanding, and the celebration of diversity. The art of hugging becomes a dynamic force that enriches the global narrative for generations to come.

In the grand finale of this chapter, we stand at the crossroads of diverse hugging customs, marveling at the symphony of connections formed through the universal language of embraces. The beauty of cultural diversity is not just acknowledged but celebrated, fostering a global community where the rich tapestry of hugging traditions becomes a testament to the shared heartbeat of humanity.

In "Hug Me Close: The Art of Hugging," Chapter 6 invites readers to embark on a global journey of understanding, embracing the richness of cultural diversity in hugging etiquettes and fostering connections that transcend borders with respect and appreciation.

CHAPTER SEVEN

Hugging in the Digital Age

As we delve into the final chapter of "Hug Me Close: The Art of Hugging," we navigate the uncharted territories of the digital era, where screens mediate our interactions, and connections transcend physical boundaries. Chapter 7 explores the evolution of hugging in the digital age, uncovering how technology transforms the art of embracing in ways both unique and unprecedented.

The Rise of Virtual Hugs:

In a world where physical distance can be vast, virtual hugs emerge as a creative and heartfelt way to bridge the gap. This section delves into the realm of emojis, GIFs, and virtual embraces, exploring how these digital expressions have become a modern language for conveying affection across screens. Readers will discover the power of virtual hugs in maintaining connections, even when physical presence is not possible.

In an era where the expanse of physical distance often separates loved ones, a new form of emotional connection has emerged – the virtual hug. In this age of digital communication, where screens serve as bridges between hearts, the language of affection has evolved into a rich tapestry of emojis, GIFs, and virtual embraces. This section delves into the fascinating realm of these digital expressions, exploring how they have become a poignant and creative means of maintaining connections across vast distances.

Emojis, those small, expressive icons that have become integral to our online conversations, play a crucial role in the rise of virtual hugs. From the classic smiling face with open arms to the cozy heartwarming emoticons, these symbols transcend language barriers and convey a universal message of warmth and care. The simplicity of a well-chosen emoji can speak volumes, allowing individuals to express emotions that words may struggle to capture.

GIFs, short animated images, add an extra layer of dynamism to virtual hugs. These moving pictures, often accompanied by heartwarming messages, create a sense of presence that goes beyond static text. The virtual hug GIFs, depicting cartoon characters or real-life moments of embracing, manage to evoke a genuine feeling of connection, making it almost tangible through the screen.

The art of sending virtual hugs extends beyond mere symbols and animations; it's about cultivating a modern language for conveying affection. In a world where physical touch may not always be feasible, the digital realm offers a space for emotional intimacy. The virtual hug transcends geographical boundaries, allowing friends, family, and even acquaintances to share moments of support, empathy, and joy.

What makes virtual hugs so powerful is their ability to maintain connections when physical presence is not possible. Whether it's consoling a friend going through a tough time or celebrating a milestone from afar, the virtual hug provides a comforting reassurance that emotions can be shared and understood, even through the pixels of a screen.

As the world continues to navigate the challenges of physical separation, the rise of virtual hugs exemplifies the resilience of human connections. These digital expressions have become more than just symbols on a screen; they are a testament to our innate need for connection and the adaptability of human emotion in the face of technological evolution. In a society where distances can be vast, the virtual hug stands as a reminder that, no matter how far apart we may be, our ability to convey love and support remains ever-present in the virtual embrace.

Embracing the Emoji:

Emojis have become an integral part of our digital communication, offering a visual language to express emotions. This part of the chapter explores how emojis, particularly the hugging ones, contribute to the digital landscape of affection. Readers will gain insights into the nuances of using virtual hugs to convey emotions ranging from joy and support to empathy and warmth.

In the ever-evolving landscape of digital communication, emojis have emerged as powerful tools to convey emotions in a concise and expressive manner. Among these symbols, the hugging emojis stand out as a unique and universal way to communicate affection, empathy, and support. This chapter delves into the fascinating world of hugging emojis, exploring their nuances and the profound impact they have on our digital interactions.

The Universality of Hugging Emojis:

One remarkable aspect of hugging emojis is their universality. Regardless of cultural and linguistic differences, the visual representation of a hug is universally understood. This simple yet profound gesture transcends language barriers, making it a potent means of connecting with others on a deeper emotional level.

Expressing Joy and Celebration:

Hugging emojis play a crucial role in expressing joy and celebration in digital conversations. Whether it's a congratulatory message, a birthday wish, or a shared success, the virtual hug adds a layer of warmth and sincerity to the text. It transforms a mere message into a heartfelt expression of shared happiness, creating a sense of camaraderie in the digital space.

Conveying Support and Empathy:

In times of sadness, distress, or hardship, hugging emojis become powerful tools for conveying support and empathy. A virtual hug sent during moments of vulnerability can provide comfort and reassurance, creating a digital space where individuals feel understood and cared for. The visual representation of a hug serves as a reminder that, even in the virtual world, one is not alone.

Nuances of Digital Affection:

As the digital landscape continues to shape the way we communicate, the nuances of conveying affection through hugging emojis become increasingly important. Understanding when and how to use these symbols adds depth to our online interactions. From a gentle embrace to a hearty squeeze, the variety of hugging emojis allows users to tailor their expressions of affection to the specific context and relationship.

The Evolution of Hugging Emojis:

As technology advances, so too do the ways in which we express ourselves digitally. The chapter explores the evolution of hugging emojis, considering how new variations and designs reflect changing social norms and communication trends. From classic yellow smileys to more detailed and diverse representations, the evolution of hugging emojis mirrors the ever-expanding range of emotions we seek to convey in the digital realm.

Hugging Across Time Zones:

With friendships and relationships spanning across time zones, digital communication becomes a lifeline. This section examines the challenges and opportunities presented by hugging in a digital world, where video calls, voice messages, and virtual embraces become essential tools in maintaining connections despite geographical distances. Readers will learn how technology acts as a conduit for emotional closeness in the face of physical separation.

In a globalized world where friendships and relationships transcend geographical boundaries, the challenge of connecting across time zones becomes an intricate dance of digital communication. This section unravels the complexities of maintaining relationships when physical proximity is not an option, exploring the role of video calls, voice messages, and virtual embraces as essential tools for bridging the gap.

The digital realm offers both challenges and opportunities when it comes to hugging across time zones. The distance, both temporal and spatial, adds a layer of complexity to communication, but it also provides an arena for innovation and creativity in expressing emotions. Video calls, in particular, emerge as a lifeline, allowing individuals to see and hear their loved ones in real-time, transcending the limitations of written text.

Voice messages, with their nuanced tone and personal touch, become a unique form of hugging through technology. In a world where written words may fall short in conveying the depth of emotions, the warmth and sincerity captured in a voice message serve as a powerful bridge, connecting hearts across time zones.

Virtual embraces, manifested through emojis and GIFs, take on a heightened significance in the context of hugging across time zones. These digital expressions not only convey emotions but also serve as a symbolic representation of the intangible connection between individuals separated by hours or even days. The simplicity of a well-timed virtual hug can dissolve the temporal gap, making the distance feel less formidable.

Technology acts as a conduit for emotional closeness, offering a lifeline to those navigating relationships across time zones. The ability to share everyday moments, celebrate milestones, or provide comfort through digital means becomes a testament to the adaptability of human connection. The challenges posed by distance are met with the resilience of communication tools that facilitate a sense of presence, even when physical togetherness is unattainable.

As readers navigate the intricacies of hugging across time zones, they will discover the transformative power of technology in maintaining and nourishing relationships. In a world where temporal differences can create a sense of disconnection, the tools of digital communication become the threads weaving a tapestry of emotional intimacy, proving that despite the challenges, love and connection know no bounds.

The Impact of Social Media on Hugging Culture:

Social media platforms have redefined the way we connect, share, and express affection. This part of the chapter explores how social media influences hugging culture, from the public display of affection through photos to the creation of online communities centered around shared interests and support. Readers will gain insights into the evolving dynamics of digital hugging within the social media landscape.

Social media has become an integral part of our daily lives, reshaping the way we communicate and express ourselves. In this chapter, we delve into the impact of social media on hugging culture, examining how these platforms influence the public display of affection, create virtual communities, and contribute to the evolving dynamics of digital hugging.

Public Display of Affection (PDA) in the Digital Age:

Social media platforms provide a virtual stage for the public display of affection, and hugging culture has found its place in this digital spotlight. Users share moments of intimacy, celebrations, and connections through visual content, often accompanied by hugging emojis or captions expressing warmth and closeness. The digital realm allows for the dissemination of affectionate gestures on a global scale, fostering a sense of connection among users despite physical distances.

Hugging Emojis as Social Currency:

Within the context of social media, hugging emojis serve as a form of social currency. Users leverage these symbols to express support, solidarity, and camaraderie in the digital space. Whether responding to a friend's achievement, consoling someone in times of difficulty, or simply sharing moments of joy, the strategic use of hugging emojis enhances the emotional depth of online interactions.

Creating Virtual Communities:

Social media has given rise to virtual communities centered around shared interests, causes, or support networks. Hugging culture extends beyond individual expressions of affection, manifesting in the formation of online groups where members share and receive virtual hugs. These communities become digital safe spaces, fostering a sense of belonging and understanding that transcends geographical boundaries.

Influencers and Trends:

In the realm of social media, influencers play a pivotal role in shaping trends and cultural expressions. The chapter explores how influencers leverage hugging culture to connect with their audience on a personal level. From scripted hugging poses to candid moments captured on camera, influencers contribute to the normalization and popularization of digital hugging, influencing a wider audience and shaping the cultural landscape.

Challenges and Controversies:

While social media has undoubtedly facilitated the spread of hugging culture, it also presents challenges and controversies. The chapter examines instances where digital affection may be perceived as performative or insincere, exploring the blurred lines between genuine expressions of emotion and the curated nature of online content. Additionally, the potential for misinterpretation and the commodification of intimacy raise questions about the authenticity of hugging culture in the social media era.

Navigating the Challenges of Digital Hugging:

While the digital age opens new avenues for hugging, it also presents unique challenges.

This section discusses the potential pitfalls of relying on digital embraces, such as misinterpretation of emotions and the need for balance between virtual and physical connections. Readers will learn to navigate the complexities of digital hugging with awareness and mindfulness.

In the era of digital communication, where hugs take on virtual forms, a new set of challenges emerges alongside the opportunities for connection. This section delves into the potential pitfalls of relying on digital embraces, emphasizing the importance of awareness and mindfulness in navigating the complexities of expressing emotions through screens.

One notable challenge in the realm of digital hugging is the risk of misinterpretation. While emojis, GIFs, and other virtual expressions strive to convey emotions, the inherent limitations of these symbols can lead to misunderstandings. Readers will explore the subtle nuances that might get lost in translation, and the importance of clarifying intentions in the digital landscape to avoid potential emotional misfires.

Another aspect to consider is the balance between virtual and physical connections. As digital hugging becomes a prevalent means of expressing affection, the need for genuine, in-person interactions remains essential. This section will guide readers in recognizing the potential pitfalls of overreliance on digital embraces, encouraging a thoughtful approach that maintains a balance between the convenience of technology and the authenticity of face-to-face connections.

Furthermore, the transient nature of digital communication poses a challenge in sustaining deep emotional connections. In a world inundated with messages and notifications, the profound impact of a virtual hug can sometimes be diluted. Readers will discover strategies for fostering meaningful digital connections, ensuring that the gestures of care and support remain impactful amid the noise of the digital landscape.

Navigating the challenges of digital hugging requires a heightened sense of awareness and mindfulness. This section aims to equip readers with the tools to read between the lines of digital expressions, fostering a deeper understanding of emotions conveyed through screens. It encourages a holistic approach that acknowledges the significance of both virtual and physical connections, promoting a balanced and meaningful engagement in the realm of digital affection.

As readers explore the potential pitfalls and solutions presented in this section, they will gain valuable insights into the art of digital hugging, learning to navigate the complexities with sensitivity and intentionality. In a world where technology continues to shape the way we express emotions, the ability to navigate these challenges becomes paramount for fostering genuine and lasting connections.

The Future of Hugging in a Technological World:

As we conclude our exploration of hugging in the digital age, we ponder the future of this age-old art in a rapidly advancing technological world. The chapter speculates on the potential innovations and advancements that may further enhance our ability to connect emotionally, exploring the exciting possibilities that lie ahead in the realm of digital hugging.

As we stand at the crossroads of human connection and technological innovation, the future of hugging takes on a fascinating trajectory. In this exploration of the digital age, we contemplate the evolution of this timeless expression of emotion and the potential advancements that await us in the world of technological hugging.

One intriguing avenue for the future is the development of haptic technology. Imagine a world where virtual reality (VR) and augmented reality (AR) seamlessly integrate with haptic feedback systems, allowing individuals to experience the sensation of a warm embrace even when physically apart. These haptic hugs could simulate the pressure, warmth, and heartbeat associated with a genuine human embrace, creating a profound sense of connection across vast distances.

Furthermore, the advent of advanced robotics promises to revolutionize the way we perceive and engage in hugging. Humanoid robots equipped with sophisticated sensors and responsive materials may become our digital companions, offering comforting hugs on demand. These robotic entities could be designed to adapt their embrace based on the emotional cues received, providing a customized and empathetic hugging experience.

As artificial intelligence continues to advance, we can anticipate the emergence of AI-driven virtual companions that excel in understanding and responding to our emotional needs. These digital entities might offer virtual hugs through personalized avatars, incorporating machine learning to adapt their hugging style to match individual preferences and emotional states.

The rise of social virtual reality spaces could redefine the landscape of digital hugging. Imagine stepping into a virtual world where friends and loved ones gather, transcending physical limitations to share genuine hugs in a simulated environment. With the help of immersive technologies, individuals could feel the presence of their loved ones and experience the joy of hugging, albeit in a virtual realm.

However, as we embrace these exciting possibilities, ethical considerations must be forefront in our minds. Questions regarding privacy, consent, and the impact of technology on genuine human connection become increasingly important. Striking a balance between technological innovation and preserving the authenticity of human interactions will be paramount in shaping the future of hugging in our technologically-driven world.

In conclusion, the future of hugging in a technological world holds promises of profound connection and emotional intimacy. From haptic experiences and robotic companions to AI-driven virtual hugs, the possibilities are vast. As we navigate this uncharted territory, let us ensure that the essence of human connection remains at the heart of our innovations, creating a future where technology enhances, rather than replaces, the timeless art of hugging.

Balancing the Digital and Physical:

The final part of the chapter advocates for a balanced approach to hugging in the digital age. While technology offers unprecedented ways to connect, it cannot replace the depth and richness of physical embraces. Readers are encouraged to strike a harmonious balance, leveraging the benefits of digital hugging while cherishing the irreplaceable warmth of face-to-face connections.

As we delve into the intricate dance between the digital and physical realms of hugging, it becomes imperative to advocate for a balanced approach that acknowledges the unique strengths of each. While technology opens up unprecedented avenues for connection, it is crucial to recognize that the depth and richness of physical embraces remain unparalleled. In this final segment, we advocate for a harmonious balance, urging readers to navigate the digital age with a thoughtful blend of innovation and tradition.

The digital landscape has undeniably transformed the way we express affection and maintain connections. Virtual hugs, conveyed through screens and devices, bridge geographical gaps and offer a semblance of closeness in an increasingly interconnected world. The convenience of sending an emoji hug or sharing a heartfelt message through digital platforms has become an integral part of modern communication.

However, as we embrace these technological marvels, it is paramount to remember that the screen can never replicate the authenticity of a physical embrace. The warmth, the subtle nuances of touch, and the emotional resonance embedded in a genuine hug are elements that defy digital replication. In advocating for balance, we encourage readers to cherish and prioritize face-to-face connections, appreciating the irreplaceable value of physical presence.

Finding equilibrium in the digital age involves a conscious effort to blend the convenience of virtual hugs with the profound significance of in-person embraces. Striking this balance requires mindfulness and an awareness of the emotional depth that physical connections bring. While technology facilitates communication, it is the tangible, sensory experience of hugging that enriches our emotional well-being.

As we navigate the future of hugging, let us not lose sight of the timeless beauty inherent in physical touch. In a world where digital connections abound, the authenticity of face-to-face encounters becomes a treasure to be safeguarded. Readers are encouraged to embrace technology for its ability to augment our connections but to never forget the essence of a heartfelt, physical hug.

In essence, the chapter concludes with a call to action — a call to embrace both the digital and physical dimensions of hugging. By striking a harmonious balance between the two, we can harness the benefits of technology while preserving the sacred intimacy of in-person connections. In doing so, we ensure that the art of hugging continues to thrive in a world where the digital and physical coexist, complementing each other in a dance of human connection.

In "Hug Me Close: The Art of Hugging," Chapter 7 provides a thought-provoking exploration of how the age-old art of hugging adapts, evolves, and thrives in the digital landscape, inviting readers to embrace the opportunities and challenges presented by technology in fostering connections in the 21st century.

CHAPTER EIGHT

Conclusion: The Enduring Warmth of Hugs

In the final embrace of "Hug Me Close: The Art of Hugging," we bask in the timeless warmth that hugs bring to our lives. This concluding chapter is a heartfelt reflection on the profound impact of embracing the art of hugging as a lifelong practice—a practice that extends far beyond the pages of this exploration.

The Unspoken Language of the Heart:

Hugs, we discover, are the unspoken language of the heart, transcending words and cultural boundaries. Whether shared between family members, friends, or strangers, the enduring warmth of a hug communicates a universal message of love, understanding, and connection. This chapter invites readers to reflect on the moments in their lives when a simple embrace spoke volumes, stitching together the fabric of their memories and relationships.

In the tapestry of human connection, hugs emerge as the unspoken language of the heart, weaving threads of emotion that transcend the limitations of words and cultural divides. Whether exchanged between family members, friends, or even strangers, the enduring warmth of a hug carries a universal message—a silent symphony of love, understanding, and connection. This chapter serves as an invitation for readers to embark on a reflective journey, urging them to ponder the moments in their lives when a simple embrace spoke volumes, delicately stitching together the fabric of their memories and relationships.

Hugs possess a unique ability to convey the profound sentiments that words often struggle to capture. In the arms of a loved one, the worries of the world can melt away, and a shared hug can bridge gaps in communication that words might fail to traverse. It is a nonverbal dance of empathy, a comforting embrace that communicates understanding, support, and a shared humanity.

This unspoken language extends beyond the boundaries of familiarity, allowing even strangers to connect on a profound level. In a single hug, we acknowledge a shared experience, a collective understanding of the human condition. It is a universal currency of compassion, a gesture that knows no linguistic barriers and speaks directly to the heart.

The chapter encourages readers to reflect on the moments when a hug became the eloquent expression of emotions. Whether it was a hug of solace during a challenging time, a jubilant embrace celebrating shared success, or a comforting hug offered in silence, each instance contributes to the rich tapestry of our lives.

As we explore the uncharted territories of our emotional landscapes, we find that the unspoken language of the heart is a powerful force that shapes the contours of our relationships. It is the glue that binds us together, fostering a sense of belonging and shared humanity. This chapter serves as a reminder that, in the silent eloquence of a hug, we discover a universal language that transcends cultural boundaries and speaks directly to the soul, leaving an indelible mark on the canvas of our memories and relationships.

The Healing Power of Hugs:

Throughout our journey, we explored the therapeutic dimensions of hugs—their ability to heal, to provide solace, and to foster emotional well-being. In this conclusion, we emphasize the lasting impact that intentional, compassionate hugs can have on our mental, emotional, and even physical health. Hugs, it seems, are not only an art but a source of enduring comfort and healing.

In the pages of our exploration, we ventured into the therapeutic dimensions of hugs—delving into their profound ability to heal, to offer solace, and to nurture emotional well-being. As we conclude this journey, it becomes evident that hugs are not merely an art but a profound source of enduring comfort and healing. In this final reflection, we underscore the lasting impact that intentional, compassionate hugs can have on our mental, emotional, and even physical health.

The healing power of hugs is rooted in their ability to transcend the boundaries between mind and body. Numerous studies have illuminated the physiological effects of hugs, such as the release of oxytocin—the "love hormone"—which contributes to a sense of bonding and reduces stress. These simple yet profound gestures have the capacity to lower blood pressure, alleviate anxiety, and elevate mood, offering a holistic approach to well-being.

Emotionally, hugs provide a sanctuary where individuals can find solace and support. They act as a balm for wounds that may not be visible, offering a tangible expression of care and understanding. In times of distress, a compassionate embrace can communicate empathy and provide a sense of security, creating a healing space where emotional burdens can be shared and alleviated.

Mentally, the act of hugging nurtures a sense of connection and belonging. It fosters a positive psychological environment, reinforcing the notion that we are not alone in our struggles. The power of a comforting hug lies in its ability to validate emotions and strengthen interpersonal bonds, creating a foundation for resilience and mental well-being.

As we reflect on the healing power of hugs, it becomes clear that these simple gestures are far more than a customary greeting or a fleeting moment of connection. They are intentional acts of compassion that ripple through the fabric of our lives, leaving a lasting imprint on our health and relationships.

In conclusion, this journey through the therapeutic dimensions of hugs encourages us to recognize and embrace the significance of intentional, compassionate touch. Hugs are not only an ancient art but a timeless source of comfort, healing, and connection. Let us carry forward the understanding that, in the embrace of a hug, we find not only solace for the soul but a pathway to enduring well-being.

Promoting Well-being Through Hugging:

The art of hugging is not merely a practice; it's a pathway to enhanced well-being. This chapter encourages readers to integrate the act of hugging into their daily lives, recognizing its power to reduce stress, strengthen relationships, and contribute to a more positive mental state. As we conclude our exploration, we extend an invitation to make hugging a conscious part of self-care—an enduring commitment to one's own emotional health.

In our journey through the intricate tapestry of hugging, we've uncovered that this art is not merely a practice; it serves as a profound pathway to enhanced well-being. As we draw the curtain on our exploration, this chapter extends an invitation to readers, urging them to embrace the transformative potential of hugging in their daily lives. Recognizing its power to reduce stress, strengthen relationships, and contribute to a more positive mental state, we encourage the integration of hugging as a conscious part of self-care—a steadfast commitment to one's own emotional health.

Hugging, it seems, is more than a simple physical gesture. It is a therapeutic ritual that has the potential to alleviate the burdens of the day, offering a respite from the demands of modern life. Research has consistently highlighted the stress-reducing benefits of hugs, as they trigger the release of oxytocin, a hormone associated with bonding and relaxation. By incorporating hugs into our routines, we can create pockets of calm amidst the chaos, promoting emotional resilience and well-being.

The relational aspect of hugging is equally significant. In the embrace of a hug, connections are strengthened, and a sense of belonging is reinforced. Whether shared with friends, family, or even acquaintances, hugging fosters a positive atmosphere of trust and support. By making hugs a deliberate part of our interactions, we contribute to the cultivation of meaningful relationships, fortifying the social fabric that sustains our emotional health.

The act of hugging also holds the power to shape our mental landscape. As we engage in this tactile expression of care, we pave the way for a more positive and optimistic mindset. The simplicity of a hug can uplift spirits, offering a tangible reminder that we are not alone in our journey toward well-being.

As we conclude this exploration, we extend an invitation to make hugging a conscious and intentional element of self-care. Let us embrace the idea that in the warmth of a hug, we find a sanctuary for our well-being—an oasis where stress dissipates, connections flourish, and mental resilience is nurtured. By recognizing the art of hugging as a powerful contributor to enhanced well-being, we embark on a journey of self-care that is both timeless and transformative.

Creating a More Connected World:

In a world that sometimes feels divided, hugging stands as a testament to our shared humanity. The conclusion underscores the role of hugging in fostering connection and compassion, advocating for a more connected world where the simple act of embracing becomes a bridge between hearts. Readers are encouraged to be ambassadors of this warmth, spreading the ripple effect of kindness through the art of hugging.

In a world that can often feel fragmented and divided, the practice of hugging emerges as a powerful testament to our shared humanity. As we bring our exploration to a close, this conclusion shines a light on the pivotal role of hugging in fostering connection and compassion. It advocates for a more connected world where the simple act of embracing becomes a bridge between hearts, transcending barriers and building bridges of understanding. Readers are encouraged to become ambassadors of this warmth, spreading the ripple effect of kindness through the art of hugging.

In the tapestry of human experience, hugging is a universal language that speaks to our common desire for connection and understanding. It disregards boundaries, be they geographical, cultural, or ideological, and in the tender embrace, we find a shared ground that unites us all. This chapter celebrates the potential of hugging to mend the fractures in our social fabric, promoting a world where empathy and compassion prevail.

As readers journey through these pages, they are invited to reflect on their own role in creating a more connected world. The simple, yet profound, act of hugging serves as a catalyst for positive change, inspiring individuals to break down the walls that separate us and embrace the beauty of our shared humanity.

The invitation is extended to be conscious architects of connection, recognizing the transformative power of hugging in daily interactions. By becoming emissaries of warmth and understanding, readers can contribute to a ripple effect that extends far beyond individual embraces. The art of hugging, when shared intentionally and authentically, becomes a force that binds communities, transcends differences, and fosters a sense of belonging.

In conclusion, let us embark on a collective journey toward a more connected world—one where the simple, genuine act of hugging becomes a shared language of kindness. Through our individual efforts, we can contribute to a global movement, weaving a tapestry of compassion that bridges the gaps between hearts. As ambassadors of warmth, readers are encouraged to carry the spirit of hugging into their daily lives, creating a ripple effect that has the potential to transform our world into a more connected and compassionate place for all.

Embracing Hugging as a Lifelong Practice:

As we bid farewell to the pages of "Hug Me Close," this chapter serves as a gentle reminder that the art of hugging is not confined to the covers of a book but is a lifelong practice. Readers are invited to carry the lessons learned into their daily lives, weaving the threads of hugging into the very fabric of their existence. Through intentional embraces, they can contribute to a world that thrives on empathy, understanding, and the enduring warmth that hugging imparts.

As we turn the final pages of "Hug Me Close," it is not merely a conclusion but a prelude to a lifelong practice. This chapter serves as a gentle reminder that the art of hugging is not confined to the covers of a book; rather, it is an ever-evolving, lifelong journey. Readers are invited to carry the lessons learned within these pages into their daily lives, weaving the threads of hugging into the very fabric of their existence. Through intentional embraces, they can contribute to a world that thrives on empathy, understanding, and the enduring warmth that hugging imparts.

The embrace is not a fleeting moment but a timeless practice that holds the potential to shape the course of our lives. As readers navigate the chapters of their personal stories, they are encouraged to embrace the art of hugging as a constant companion—a source of solace, connection, and joy.

In weaving hugging into the daily tapestry of existence, individuals become architects of warmth and compassion. The practice extends beyond the pages of this book, becoming an integral part of their interactions with family, friends, colleagues, and even strangers. Through intentional embraces, readers have the power to create a ripple effect that transcends the boundaries of their personal lives, contributing to a culture of empathy and understanding.

The lessons learned from "Hug Me Close" are not confined to the theoretical; they are an invitation to action. Each hug, given with intention and authenticity, becomes a brushstroke in the portrait of a life well-lived—one characterized by meaningful connections and shared moments of tenderness.

As readers bid farewell to this exploration, they are reminded that the art of hugging is not a one-time engagement but a lifelong journey. It is an ongoing commitment to infuse their lives with the healing and connecting power of embraces. By embracing hugging as a lifelong practice, readers can play a part in shaping a world where the warmth of human connection prevails, one hug at a time.

A Heartfelt Farewell: In bidding farewell to "Hug Me Close: The Art of Hugging," we express gratitude for the shared journey. May the lessons learned within these pages inspire a world where hugging is not just an art form but a universal language—a language that speaks of love, compassion, and the enduring warmth that binds us all.

As we tenderly bid farewell to the pages of "Hug Me Close: The Art of Hugging," we express profound gratitude for the shared journey. The lessons learned within these pages have been more than words on paper;

they have been a shared exploration of the profound and transformative power of human connection.

May the echoes of our shared exploration resonate in the hearts of readers, inspiring a world where hugging is not merely an art form but a universal language—a language that speaks of love, compassion, and the enduring warmth that binds us all. In each embrace, may the lessons of this journey be felt, and may the ripple effect of intentional hugs extend far beyond the covers of this book.

As we part ways, let the spirit of hugging linger in our lives—a gentle reminder of the beauty that unfolds when hearts connect. In the dance of each hug, may we find a reflection of our shared humanity, a reminder that, despite our differences, we are bound by the common thread of the human experience.

Thank you for sharing in the exploration of "Hug Me Close." May the lessons learned guide us towards a world where the language of the heart, spoken through the simple yet profound act of hugging, becomes a beacon of light, fostering love and connection in every corner of our shared existence. Until we meet again, may your days be filled with the warmth of genuine embraces and the joy of connecting with the hearts of those around you.

May your embraces be plentiful, your connections deep, and your world forever enriched by the enduring warmth of hugs.

Epilogue

In the gentle afterglow of our exploration within the pages of "Hug Me Close: The Art of Hugging," we find ourselves at the threshold of the epilogue—a moment to reflect on the enduring echoes of warmth and connection that hugs have imprinted on our hearts.

A Tapestry of Shared Embraces: The epilogue invites readers to reflect on the myriad embraces encountered throughout the journey, recognizing that the art of hugging is not confined to chapters but woven into the tapestry of our shared human experience. Each embrace, whether virtual or physical, becomes a brushstroke in the masterpiece of our lives—a masterpiece painted with strokes of compassion, understanding, and love.

Carrying the Art Forward: As we close this chapter of exploration, the epilogue extends an invitation to carry the art of hugging forward into the vast expanse of life. Readers are encouraged to let the lessons learned guide them in creating moments of connection, understanding, and shared humanity. The book, in essence, becomes a companion for life—a reminder that in the embrace, we find a language that transcends the constraints of time and space.

A Legacy of Hugs: The epilogue gently contemplates the legacy that the art of hugging leaves behind. As readers navigate the chapters of their own stories, the book becomes a source of inspiration—an enduring guide that whispers reminders of the profound impact simple embraces can have on the human experience. In cultivating a legacy of hugs, we contribute to a world where warmth and compassion prevail.

An Invitation to Share: In its final moments, the epilogue extends an open invitation for readers to share their experiences, reflections, and newfound perspectives on hugging. Whether through personal stories, anecdotes, or the impact of embracing the art in their lives, readers are encouraged to contribute to the ongoing narrative of the shared journey.

Gratitude for the Journey: With heartfelt gratitude, the epilogue expresses appreciation for the shared odyssey. It acknowledges the beauty found in the diversity of hugs, the warmth discovered in the therapeutic power of embraces, and the interconnectedness experienced through the universal language of hugging. The book bids farewell, knowing that the art of hugging will continue to unfold in the lives of those who embraced its teachings.

As we close the cover on "Hug Me Close: The Art of Hugging," may the echoes of our shared exploration resonate in the gentle rustle of pages, reminding us that the enduring warmth of hugs is a gift to be cherished, shared, and celebrated throughout the chapters of our lives.

…..***…..